RECIPE
for a
LONG, HEALTHY LIFE

RECIPE
for a
LONG,
HEALTHY
LIFE

Adrian Joele

Copyright © 2021 by Adrian Joele.

Library of Congress Control Number: 2021919149
ISBN: Hardcover   978-1-9845-0830-0
                    Softcover   978-1-9845-0829-4
                    eBook   978-1-9845-0828-7

Print information available on the last page.

Rev. date: 10/01/2021

\

To order additional copies of this book, contact:
Xlibris
AU TFN: 1 800 844 927 (Toll Free inside Australia)
AU Local: (02) 8310 8187 (+61 2 8310 8187 from outside Australia)
www.Xlibris.com.au
Orders@Xlibris.com.au
820415

Contents

Introduction

The human potential for wellness of body and mind to enable life to be enjoyed to the full far exceeds the wildest expectations of modern society.

This book contains information, recommendations, and guidelines in order to be able to live a healthy lifestyle that is based on good nutrition and exercise, like aerobics, high-intensity aerobics, and weightlifting.

The book also describes subjects about many factors that determine good nutrition and overall health.

I haven't met anyone who does not want to have excellent health. Most of us assume that we always will. But it's a fact that many of us (doctors included) are losing our health each day.

There is overwhelming evidence that by choosing to eat the right foods, and by making simple changes in your lifestyle, you can prevent and even reverse more diseases than any doctor, hospital, and drug, or any combination of medical treatments known to man.

You should not exercise or take large doses of nutrients on a regular basis without the advice of a physician, who knows about nutrition. Nutrients and exercise can have an adverse effect on some diseases, and some nutrients can neutralize the effects of certain prescribed medications.

Generally, physicians are disease-oriented. They are pharmaceutically trained to treat diseases. They learn how the body absorbs each drug and when and how the body excretes it. They learn the side effects of drugs, and they take care to balance the benefits against any potential danger. Physicians know their drugs, and they don't hesitate to prescribe them.

Just consider the number of drugs that are taken for high blood pressure, elevated cholesterol, diabetes mellitus, arthritis, heart disease, and depression, just to name a few. As a result of the discovery and use of antibiotics in the war against infectious diseases, their philosophy in medicine has become to attack disease.

Because physicians are disease- and drug-oriented, they spent most of their time and effort trying to identify a disease process so they can prescribe a drug or treatment plan for their patients.

Yet it just makes common sense that it is much easier to maintain your health than to try to regain it after you have lost it.

Doctors want to know if you have elevated cholesterol, whether you have become diabetic, or developed hypertension. But they spend very little time trying to help the patient understand the lifestyle changes that are necessary to actually protect his or her health. Physicians are too busy treating all the disease they meet each and every day.

As a consequence of our modern lifestyle, we will give way to some type of degenerative disease sooner than we would like. However, there is also a parallel interest in finding a way to avoid what seems inevitable. Many people have quit smoking, taking up exercise, changed their diet, and in general tried to take more responsibility toward prevention of any illness.

This book can be an excellent beginning along the road to health. It is the first step in what can be a progression to a healthier and more productive life.

Chapter 1

1. A Guide to Healthy Living

Many people are in search for healthy living. But what are really the essentials for health and fitness, and how do you achieve good health and overall well-being?

When you have a closer look at the concept, it all boils down to the following four components, which are crucial for healthy living:

1. good nutrition
2. regular exercise
3. a good night sleep
4. high-quality nutritional supplementation

If we choose to make good nutrition—including supplementation—and an active lifestyle a daily habit, we could add five to fifteen healthy years to our lives.

Healthy living means keeping a balanced, healthy diet. Avoid smoking and excessive use of alcohol and toxic chemicals. Take regular exercise, have a good night sleep, and supplement your diet with high-quality nutritional supplements.

I will describe in more detail the above-mentioned four components for healthy living.

First of all, good nutrition.

The key to fitness is nutrition; we are mainly what we eat. You probably heard it before: 'You are what you eat.' Although I like a more accurate definition. It is better to say, 'You are what you can get out of your food.'

It is true that exercise, restful sleep, peace of mind, regular habits of elimination, bathing, etc. are all factors in keeping fit, but these will avail nothing if our nutrition is at fault.

It is now recognized that most common illnesses are closely associated with nutrition and arise from lack of vitamins and minerals, just as some more serious ailments, such as scurvy, rickets, anaemia, beriberi, pellagra, and nerve troubles, are equally deficiency ailments and respond to appropriate vitamin therapy.

Periodically, new and successful uses of vitamins in diseased conditions are reported in the world's medical journals, and more and more physicians are prescribing vitamins, where some fifty years ago, they prescribed drugs.

Many people wonder why the terrible epidemics which formerly ravaged the earth—typhus, yellow fever, typhoid, cholera, malaria, bubonic plague, etc.—have largely been brought under control, yet the degenerative diseases, such as heart ailments, high blood pressure, hardening of the arteries, stomach ulcers, nervous breakdowns, colitis, cataract, and kidney and liver ailments, are all on the increase.

The reason is that the plague or 'dirt' diseases spread by vermin, mosquitoes, and human contact are disappearing owing to improved methods of hygiene and sanitation.

The degenerative diseases arise primarily from man's continual tampering with natural foods, thereby depriving them of vital nutrients that nature, in her wisdom, incorporates in our foodstuffs to ensure good health.

It is a tragic fact that most people these days only begin to take an intelligent interest in their health after they have lost it. Nature requires that we cooperate with her, and we cannot escape the consequences of our refusal to do so. Good nutrition is fundamental for good health.

The human body is a complex system that requires a full spectrum of nutrients for optimal health. What do we mean by 'good nutrition'?

Good nutrition means eating the right food that contains all the right carbohydrates, protein, fat, fatty acids, vitamins, minerals, and trace elements, based on your body type.

A second factor that determines good nutrition is our body's ability to absorb the nutrients from the food that we eat. The nutrients have to be in a form that the cells can accept them, and the cells have to be in optimum condition to be able to absorb the nutrients. This is called bioavailability.

These are the keys to successful nutrition and two often overlooked facts. That is one of the reasons most nutritional supplements miss the mark. They don't address the cellular condition of the body.

You may think that regular exercise, a positive mental attitude, and applying the golden rule 'everything in moderation' are the keys to good health.

However, if you understand the damage caused by processed foods, it will motivate you to change your diet, if you are aiming for a high level of health and freedom from degenerative diseases.

Acid–Alkaline Balance

We should consume acid- and alkaline-forming foods in the right ratios. This is not hard to realize, when we know that, generally speaking, fruits and vegetables are alkaline-forming and the rest is mostly acid-forming, with a few exceptions.

You can read more about acid- and alkaline-forming foods in my article. The Australian diet contains nearly one and a half times more acid-forming food as it does alkaline-forming food. This ratio should be the other way around.

The problem with eating too much acid-forming food is that it builds up toxic waste products and is the cause of most of our health problems. A diet that contains insufficient fruit and vegetables is missing vital antioxidants, beta-carotene, vitamins, and minerals.

They are most important to prevent oxidation, caused by free radicals, which are the main cause of heart disease, stroke, cancer, and other diseases.

We also need a sufficient number of antioxidants to counteract the formation of free radicals caused by our stressful lifestyle, pollution in air and water, and malnutrition.

Oxidative stress has shown to be the root cause of over seventy chronic degenerative diseases. Every day, the DNA in each cell in your body faces about 10,000 attacks from cell-damaging forces known as free radicals, which are unstable oxygen molecules that have lost an electron. Free radicals are naturally produced as your body turns fuel to energy, but you also get them from pollution in air and water, stress, smoking, and radiation from the sun.

These volatile molecules cruise around your body, trying to stabilize themselves by stealing electrons from other molecules. When they succeed, they create still more free radicals, causing a sort of snowballing procession of damage.

Free radicals don't just occasionally pop up here and there. Up to 5 per cent of the oxygen that each cell uses is converted into free radicals. Free-radical damage is thought to play a role in the accumulation of low-density-lipoprotein (LDL) cholesterol and the lining of your artery walls.

This can lead to a narrowing of the arteries called atherosclerosis, which contributes to heart disease. And when free radicals damage DNA inside the cells, the results can be cell mutations that lead to cancer.

It is not all about nutrition; neither is it all about exercise. A balanced lifestyle is the key.

Exercise at least three times per week. Aerobics, jogging, swimming, cycling, also include weightlifting in your exercise routine, which is important for maintaining a healthy bone structure.

The key is to do the right exercise.

Aerobics are usually recommended in the weight loss industry. The more intense, the better, which is all wrong! The problem is that aerobics exercises that raise your heart rate above 120 beats per minute, which include running, rowing, swimming, cycling, and many of those fancy aerobics classes in health clubs, all strip off muscle almost as much as they strip off fat.

And as you know, muscle loss reduces your ability to burn fat and sets you up to become even fatter. Remember, muscle is the engine in which body fat is burned. You should do everything you can to maintain it for the rest of your life.

Walking is good for many health reasons; it also burns some fat and will not burn muscle. But the best exercise for fat control is wide-variety high-repetition resistance training using weights or machines.

By exercising all the muscles of your body, you burn a lot of fat. Another advantage of resistance exercise is that it increases muscle and as a result provide more muscle cells to be able to burn fat. It's a real health bargain. Another important factor is proper pace. Don't overdo it. You can't force things to happen at once. The secret to good health is consistency and steadiness. You need to have the right amounts of food and regular exercise.

The simple technique of 'deep breathing' can make a powerful contribution to feeling good and being fit and well. Our bodies need an abundance of physical and mental energy to be able to function at their best.

The energy source is food. But food is useless without oxygen, which is the key to our power. The more oxygen we deliver to our cells, the more energy we will have.

Breathing is the way we obtain oxygen, and the benefits of periodic deep breathing are enormous. However, if our breathing is shallow, we cripple the functioning of our systems. When the oxygen supply to our lungs is not sufficient, it can contribute to illnesses, both physical and mental. Posture is important for proper breathing.

The third factor of health and fitness is a good night sleep. There is nothing more beneficial than a good night sleep, and there is a great physiological need for it if the individual likes to feel refreshed and alert during the following day. Sleep is also important for your memory and learning capacity and possibly for maintaining a good immune system. But there are still many unanswered questions regarding the function of sleep.

People who are suffering from a chronic degenerative disease are under greater oxidative stress than normal. In this case, optimizers are important to use in order to support any existing nutritional program.

It's been scientifically proven that there are substantial health benefits in taking nutritional supplements. The benefits of nutritional supplements are scientifically verified over the past two years. Hundreds of scientific studies have proven that nutritional supplements can significantly reduce the risk of degenerative diseases.

Apart from the future benefits, eating well and exercising regularly to achieve health and fitness also enable us to enjoy life so much more right now!

I have developed an exercise plan that covers the basics of exercise, aerobics, weight-bearing exercises, and nutrition for athletes.

2. Nutrition: The Key to Fitness and Well-Being

If we choose good nutrition, including supplementation, and make an active lifestyle a daily habit, we could add five to fifteen healthy years to our lives.

Without science and technology, our lifespan would not have been increased as much as we experience it today. However, they would not be able to secure for us our long-term health. As Dr Myron Wentz, founder of USANA Health Sciences likes to phrase it, 'We are living too short and dying too long.'

It is true that exercise, restful sleep, peace of mind, regular habits of elimination, batching, etc. are all factors in keeping fit, but these will avail us nothing if our nutrition is at fault. Healthy living means keeping a balanced, healthy diet; avoiding smoking and excessive use of alcohol and toxic chemicals; taking regular exercise; and supplementing our diet with high-quality nutritional supplements. It is now recognized that most common illnesses are close associated with nutrition and arise from lack of vitamins and minerals.

You need the right kind of nutrients, and they need to be in balance: balanced nutrition. That's where the name of my website, Nutrobalance, comes from.

However, the nutrients have to be in a form that the cells of our body can accept them, and the cells have to be in optimum condition to be able to absorb the nutrients. This is called bioavailability. These are the keys to a successful diet and nutrition and two often overlooked facts.

Maintaining your health is much easier than trying to regain it. When you are struggling with your health, you can empower your body to fight and even reverse chronic diseases. By providing the necessary nutrients at optimal levels, your LDL cholesterol is more resistant to oxidation, your eyes have greater antioxidant protection from sunlight, and you provide optimal protection for your lungs. You increase your immune system and antioxidant defence system. You decrease the risk of developing heart disease, stroke, cancer, arthritis, diabetes, Alzheimer's, Parkinson's disease, and more. People who are suffering from a chronic degenerative disease are under greater oxidative stress than normal. In this case, optimizers are important to use in order to support any existing nutritional program.

It's been scientifically proven that there are substantial health benefits in taking nutritional supplements.

The benefits of nutritional supplements are scientifically verified over the past two years. Hundreds of scientific studies have proven that nutritional supplements can significantly reduce the risk of degenerative diseases.

The American Medical Association (AMA) now encourages all adults to supplement daily with a multiple vitamin.

Based on a landmark review of thirty-eight years of scientific evidence by Harvard researchers Dr Robert Fletcher and Dr Kathleen Fairfield, the conservative *Journal of the American Medical Association (JAMA)* has rewritten its policy guidelines regarding the use of vitamin supplements. In a striking departure from its previous anti-vitamin rhetoric, *JAMA* (19 June 2002) now recommends that, given our nutrient-poor modern diet, supplementation each day with a multiple vitamin is a prudent preventive measure against chronic disease. The researchers point out that more than 80 per cent of the American population does not consume anywhere near the five to eight servings of fruits and vegetables required each day for optimal health.

Most people simply accept the onset of arthritis, heart disease, and diabetes as inevitable results of the ageing process—the truth is, these conditions are largely preventable. Apart from the future benefits, good nutrition and exercising regularly also enable us to enjoy life so much more right now!

3. Nutrition Facts

Antioxidants are the bodyguards of your cells.

To understand nutrition, you must first understand what free radicals and antioxidants are and how they work. Picture yourself as the president, a king or queen, a movie star, or another well-known figure.

A threat to your safety could pop up at any time, and that's why you have a team of bodyguards surrounding you. If a source of danger comes your way, your bodyguards are trained to swoop in and get between you and this threat.

Your protectors are willing to suffer the consequences themselves, just to keep you from getting hurt.

Every day, the DNA in each cell in your body faces about 10,000 attacks from cell-damaging forces known as free radicals, which are unstable oxygen molecules that have lost an electron. Free radicals are naturally produced as your body turns fuel to energy, but you also get them from pollution in air and water, stress, smoking, and radiation from the sun.

These volatile molecules cruise around your body, trying to stabilize themselves by stealing electrons from other molecules. When they succeed, they create still more free radicals, causing a sort of snowballing procession of damage.

Free radicals don't just occasionally pop up here and there. Up to 5 per cent of the oxygen that each cell uses is converted into free radicals. Free-radical damage is thought to play a role in the accumulation of low-density-lipoprotein (LDL) cholesterol and the lining of your artery walls. This can lead to a narrowing of the arteries called atherosclerosis, which contributes to heart disease. And when free radicals damage DNA inside the cells, the results can be cell mutations that lead to cancer.

Free radical assaults on your eyes may lead to cataracts and macular degeneration, which are common causes of vision loss in people over fifty years of age. Researchers think that free-radical damage—also called oxidative stress—plays an important role in Alzheimer's disease. And many scientists believe that free radicals are the primary force behind ageing itself.

Free radicals can develop and quickly attack your cells faster than the blink of an eye, and unless something is immediately available to 'step in,' this free-radical free-for-all can cause irreparable damage. That's where antioxidants come in.

Remember that analogy in which you were a famous person preyed upon by harmful threats? Those bodyguards forming a human shield around you are the oxidants in your system. Every time you eat fruits, vegetables, or other antioxidant-rich foods, a flood of these protective compounds enter your bloodstream. They travel throughout your body, stepping between your body's healthy cells and the pillaging free radicals, offering up their own electrons to neutralize the free radicals and keep your cells out of harm's way.

The Big Antioxidant Nutrients

Just as your body produces free radicals, it also produces antioxidants. Some of these are enzymes created solely to squelch free radicals. But these defenders can be overwhelmed if you're under serious attack—from car exhaust or cigarette smoke, for example—and they may be insufficient to handle rising levels of free-radical attacks as you get older.

Every day, a small percentage of free radicals slip past your natural antioxidant defences, allowing them to do damage. That's why you regularly need to call in the reserves to supplement your own forces: antioxidant compounds from your diet.

There are literally hundreds of natural food compounds that act as antioxidants in your body. Though researchers are investigating new antioxidant compounds every day, most scientific study has focused on three types in particular—vitamin C and E and carotenoids.

Here are the main antioxidants with their daily required amounts:

- N-acetyl cysteine, 50–350 mg
- L-glutathione, 100–200 mg
- vitamin A, 5,000–10,000 IU
- beta-carotene, 4.5 mg
- vitamin C as these forms:

    o ascorbic acid, 2,000–10,000 mg
    o calcium ascorbate, 1,000–1,500 mg
    o magnesium ascorbate, 250–500 mg
    o ascorbyl palmitate, 250–500 mg

- vitamin E as these forms:

    o tocopherol complex, 500–660 mg
    o d-alpha-tocopheryl succinate, 400–1,200 IU
    o zinc picolinate, 10–60 mg

- selenium as these forms:

    o selenomethionine, 200–400 mcg
    o sodium selenite, 100–200 mcg
    o coenzyme Q10, 60–100 mg

The major antioxidants and their cofactors listed here are used in laboratories to successfully inhibit a wide variety of diseases and improve the vitality of people already in excellent health.

Coenzyme Q10 is used successfully to treat various oxidation conditions and is prescribed in Japan against heart disease. L-glutathione is the only antioxidant you can use as an oral supplement. Our body makes L-glutathione, but when we age, it is not enough to inhibit particular types of oxidation.

The figures for daily amounts are averages extracted from more than 500 successful studies, guided by the antioxidant use of athletes, which is effective and non-toxic. Long-term use of antioxidant supplements is still an experiment, and the safety of amounts shown here has not been confirmed.

We would recommend using not more than the lower figures for average people. According to the *Journal of the American Medical Association*, cancer is still on the rise. Dr Deva Davis and her colleagues confirmed that cancer increase is presumably the result from exposure to carcinogens in our environment, including pesticides, herbicides, chemical solvents, smoking, and industrial and auto emissions.

Smoking is the worst out of those mentioned. The damage is done mainly by oxidation, and in combination with other air pollutants, it is the cause of 33 per cent of all cancers. Being overweight follows as the next big cancer risk with 24 per cent. The American Cancer Society began a massive study in 1959 involving more than 1 million people in twenty-five American states, which ended in 1980.

The results showed that people who are 40 per cent or more overweight have higher rates of a wide variety of cancers. Many of these cancers are caused by lipid oxidation, which means excess fat molecules in your body go rancid and initiate cell damage that develops into cancer.

For the average person, pesticides prove to be a bigger cancer threat than being overweight. Cancer risk from too much body fat is much higher than all the pesticides together.

Oxidation in our body is the main cause of many forms of cancer, heart disease, atherosclerosis, adult-onset diabetes, cataracts, lung and liver disorders, and degenerative diseases of the brain and can be prevented and even reversed by the proper use of the right antioxidants.

Protection against LDL, the 'bad' cholesterol, from oxidation depends on the fat-soluble antioxidants that can get inside the LDL particles and the water-soluble antioxidants that get into the fluids surrounding the LDL. You need some of both.

The best fat-soluble antioxidants are beta-carotene, vitamin E, and coenzyme Q10.

Recent studies show that all three nutrients prevent oxidation of human LDL in vitro (in the test tube).

The result of other studies shows that the main water-soluble vitamin, vitamin C, acts synergistically to spare vitamin E stores by restoring used vitamin E to an active state.

More importantly, vitamin C prevents macrophages from absorbing LDL in the first place. In the latest study by Drs I. Jialal and S. Grundy at the University of Texas Medical Center, vitamin C prevented uptake of LDL by macrophages by 95 per cent.

That makes vitamin C your most important defence against atherosclerosis. Recent studies at the University of Texas Medical Center show that healthy individuals supplemented with vitamin E were less subject to LDL oxidation.

Epidemiological studies also show that people with high intake of beta-carotene, vitamin E, and vitamin C have a lower incidence of coronary heart disease.

A subgroup with heart disease at the start of the study already showed a 44 per cent reduction in heart attacks and death.

Excess blood sugar levels in diabetics can cause damage of arteries, eyes, kidneys, and the brain. One solution to reduce this problem is to eat less sugar. But Americans, for example, consume half a pound of sugar per day on average.

Much of the sugar added to our food is hidden as the label reads, 'Grape juice concentrate,' 'Sweetened with fruit juice,' and 'Corn syrup.' All these are just refined liquid sugars.

Health authorities neglect to advice the public that refined sugar is as big a health risk as fat. Prediabetes is epidemic in America, with all its attendant problems, like heart disease, kidney failure, blindness, and early death. Diabetic damage from sugar occurs mainly by oxidation of fat molecules to form toxic lipid peroxides.

Many recent studies show that the antioxidant vitamin E can protect diabetic animals from this damage. Complex mechanisms neutralize sugar directly and reduce peroxide formation. This works in human diabetics too. A recent study by Dr G. Paolisso at the University of Naples, Italy, gave diabetics 900 IU of vitamin

E for four months. The diabetics showed a significant reduction in blood sugar levels.

They also showed a significant increase in endogenous antioxidants, such as glutathione, indicating a reduced pressure on the body's antioxidant defence system.

'Antioxidants can save you from a lot of its damaging effects, even if you can't avoid all the sugar in your diet. There is no doubt that antioxidants play a crucial role in reducing the risk for all kinds of diseases,' says Roc Ordman, PhD, professor of chemistry and biochemistry at Beloit College in Beloit, Wisconsin. 'The published scientific evidence is simply overwhelming.'

Would you like to live a long and healthy life? If it's going to be, it's all up to you! That sounds simple, but it's a fact! Health is a matter of *choice*!

If you want to obtain optimal health from nutrition, you have to understand first how much of what you put in your body affects your health. The human body was designed with lots of care in order to transform a mixture of certain compounds that are found in nature into muscles, bones, organs, glands, and our brain. The interactions of these nutrient compounds are the hairy bags of chemical soup that we call human beings. Every time we mess around with them, they will mess around with you.

People who consume fatty burgers with nutrient-poor fries don't realize how much they are disturbing the excellent precision of nutrient use by their bodies.

Let's look at some nutritional information to make clear how that precision makes the engine of a Maserati look like a child's toy. Let's look at a good one: vitamin B12. You need only a few micrograms (millionths of a gram) of vitamin B12 each day: the RDA (recommended daily allowance) is only 2 micrograms. Your blood contains only about 5 nanograms (billionths of a gram) per litre, less than a speck of dust. Even under a microscope, you couldn't see such amount. It represents less than one part per trillion of your body weight. But if you lack that tiny speck, your total body declines into a serious disease called pernicious anaemia, which gradually destroys the myelin sheaths, which protect your nerves, leading to blindness, insanity, and death.

A second example is iodine.

A daily intake of about 50 micrograms is considered to be sufficient for most people. This amount is still so tiny that you could hardly see it on the head of a pin.

Every day, your body separates the few molecules of iodine that occur in different foods with a precision that goes far beyond the most advanced computer and transports them straight to the thyroid gland. There they convert an inert chemical called thyronine into powerful thyroid hormones. These hormones then control your energy supply, your mood, and even how well you can think.

The same applies to other micronutrients. It is still a mystery how such minute amounts of these substances can hold the keys to health, to sanity, and even to life itself. But they do, and if they are deficient in your food, you are asking for disease.

We need a daily dose of a precise mix of fifty-nine nutrients for optimal bodily function from the following nutrition data.

Elements required in large amounts daily: oxygen, carbon, hydrogen, sulphur, nitrogen

Elements required in medium amounts daily: calcium, phosphorus, magnesium, sodium, potassium, chloride

Elements required in small amounts daily: iron, manganese, chromium, fluoride, arsenic, germanium, zinc, silicon, selenium, molybdenum, boron, copper, cobalt, iodine, nickel, tin

Vitamins (common form names): A (retinol), B3 (niacin, niacinamide), B12 (cobalamin), C (ascorbic acid), K (phylloquinone), B1 (thiamine), B5 (pantothenic acid), folic acid, D (calciferol), B2 (riboflavin), B6 (pyridoxine), biotin, E (d-alpha tocopherol)

Cofactors (common form names): choline, para-aminobenzoic acid (PABA), pyrroloquinoline quinone (PQQ), inositol, bioflavonoids, coenzyme Q10

Essential amino acids: isoleucine, methionine, tryptophan, histidine, leucine, phenylalanine, valine, taurine, lysine, threonine, arginine

The following are conditionally essential:

Essential fatty acids: linoleic acid, linolenic acid

From some, you need a lot; others you need only tiny amounts. But they all have to be provided in the correct amounts. The first five, which you need in large quantities, are plentiful present in foods and in the air we breathe, so supply is not often a problem.

The remaining fifty-four nutrients we need in medium or small quantities and are less readily available in the environment. More important, they may be deficient or entirely absent in any of the degraded foods that we now find in most of our food supply. We know that thirteen vitamins, twenty-two minerals, six cofactors, eight amino acids (plus three more in certain circumstances), and two essential fatty acids are required for optimal bodily function.

All these essential substances interact with one another in precise synergy to produce, maintain, and renew your body. If one is missing or in short supply, the functions of all the others are impaired. Although the comprehension 'essential' of cofactors is still controversial, they are included because recent evidence all points in that direction.

The meaning of the word *essential* in science means as follows:

a) The nutrients have to be present in adequate amounts, or function is impaired.
b) The body can't make the nutrients or can't make enough of them for normal tissue function.
c) You have to get them from your diet.

If you can't get them from your diet, you have to supplement them from a high-quality source.

I hope these dietary guidelines will help you on your way to a healthy life.

If we choose to make good nutrition, including supplementation, and an active lifestyle a daily habit, we could add five to fifteen healthy years to our lives.

Without science and technology, our lifespan would not have been increased as much as we experience it today. However, they would not be able to secure for us our long-term health.

As Dr Myron Wentz, founder of USANA Health Sciences, likes to phrase it, 'We are living too short and dying too long.'

Healthy living means keeping a balanced, healthy diet; avoiding smoking and excessive use of alcohol and toxic chemicals; taking regular exercise; and supplementing our diet with high-quality nutritional supplements. However, the nutrients have to be in a form that the cells of our body can accept them, and the cells have to be in optimum condition to be able to absorb the nutrients. This is called bioavailability.

These are the keys to successful nutrition and two often overlooked facts.

Maintaining your health is much easier than trying to regain it. When you are struggling with your health, you can empower your body to fight and even reverse chronic diseases.

By providing the necessary nutrients at optimal levels, your LDL cholesterol is more resistant to oxidation. Your eyes have greater antioxidant protection from sunlight, and you provide optimal protection for your lungs.

You increase your immune system and antioxidant defence system.

You decrease the risk of developing heart disease, stroke, cancer, arthritis, diabetes, Alzheimer's, Parkinson's disease, and more. People who are suffering from a chronic degenerative disease are under greater oxidative stress than normal. In this case, optimizers are important to use in order to support any existing nutritional program.

It's been scientifically proven that there are substantial health benefits in taking nutritional supplements. The benefits of nutritional supplements are scientifically verified over the past two years. Hundreds of scientific studies have proved that nutritional supplements can significantly reduce the risk of degenerative diseases.

The American Medical Association (AMA) now encourages all adults to supplement daily with a multiple vitamin. Based on a landmark review of thirty-eight years of scientific evidence by Harvard researchers Dr Robert Fletcher and Dr Kathleen Fairfield, the conservative *Journal of the American Medical Association (JAMA)* has rewritten its policy guidelines regarding the use of vitamin supplements. In a striking departure from its previous anti-vitamin rhetoric, *JAMA* (19 June 2002) now recommends that, given our nutrient-poor modern diet, supplementation each day with a multiple vitamin is a prudent preventive measure against chronic disease. The researchers point out that more than 80 per cent of the American population does not consume anywhere near the five to eight servings of fruits and vegetables required each day for optimal health. Most people simply accept the onset of arthritis, heart disease, and diabetes as inevitable results of the ageing process—the truth is, these conditions are largely preventable.

Apart from the future benefits, eating well and exercising regularly also enable us to enjoy life so much more right now!

Macronutrients

Macronutrients should take up the largest portion of your diet. This category of nutrients include carbohydrates, protein, and fat. Your body uses macronutrients for energy, growth, and repair.

Different types of macronutrients do different things for your body, so it is important to get variety in your daily diet so that you get the right types of each class of macronutrient.

Carbohydrates

Carbohydrates come in two forms: simple and complex.

Simple carbohydrates are sugars that don't need to be broken down further, so the body can use them for quick boosts of energy. Honey, maple syrup, soda, cookies, candy, table sugar, and cakes are all sources of simple sugars, but since they are also high in calories, they should only be eaten occasionally.

Instead, it is important to eat healthy sources of simple sugars, like fruit and fat-free or low-fat milk. These alternatives to sugary sweets offer vitamins, minerals, and fibre as well.

Complex carbohydrates are larger, digest more slowly, and provide longer-lasting energy. Foods like bread, pasta, rice, oatmeal, corn, and starchy vegetables (like potatoes and carrots) contain the highest amounts. Sources you should choose most often are vegetables, beans, and whole-grain, high-fibre breads and cereals. The right carbohydrates are either complex carbohydrate or fibre and generally supply additional healthy trace elements and phytonutrients as well as energy and should have a low glycaemic index.

The glycaemic index is a way of measuring the rate at which carbohydrates are broken down and appear in the blood as simple sugars. Those foods that result in a rapid rise in blood sugar often have a high glycaemic index. Carbohydrates that are broken down slowly and cause only a moderate controlled increase in blood sugar often have a low glycaemic index. Some carbohydrates fall in between.

High-glycaemic foods provide quick energy, but it is usually short-lived, and hunger soon returns. This crash stimulates many energy responses in our body chemistry, stressing our organs.

Most convenience foods and many meal replacements and diet products on the market today are high-glycaemic.

Low-glycaemic foods provide greater satiety and sustained energy. By virtue of their slow digestion and absorption, low-glycaemic foods can help control appetite and delay hunger.

Protein

A healthy diet includes a variety of high-quality protein sources, including complete proteins, which contain all the essential amino acids. Protein is what makes up bodily tissues, like the muscles, skin, and organs. When you eat food containing protein, your digestive system breaks it down into smaller parts called amino acids. These amino acids are later used by the body to build and repair cells and tissues.

The two main sources of protein are animal products like meat, milk, fish, and eggs and vegetable products like beans, nuts, seeds, and soy. To make sure you get all the essential amino acids, it's important to eat a wide variety of these protein-rich foods, such as lean meat, fish, fat-free and low-fat dairy products, eggs, nuts, seeds, and beans.

Fats

Surprisingly, some fat is good for you! Your body needs it for proper brain development, like omega-3 and omega-6, to bring certain vitamins through the brain barrier.

There are two types of fat: saturated and unsaturated. Beneficial fats are high in essential fatty acid and low in saturated fatty acid. Unsaturated fat is found in fish like salmon and tuna, nuts, seeds, avocados, and most vegetable oils.

Most of the fat that you eat should come from these foods. Saturated fat may increase your risk of heart disease. It is important to limit the amount you consume. No more than 10 per cent of your total daily calories should be derived from saturated fat. It is found in food that come from animals, like red meat, butter, cheese, milk (except fat-free), and ice cream. Coconut and palm oils are also high in saturated fat and can be found in many store-bought baked foods.

The Importance of a Low-Fat, High-Fibre Diet

Diets low in saturated fat and cholesterol and rich in fruits and vegetables and grain products that contain some type of fibre, particularly soluble fibre, have many health benefits. Unfortunately, the normal diet in today's society includes only one-half or two-thirds of the fibre necessary for optimal health. The positive impact of a high fibre diet is increased when there is a concurrent reduction in the amount of saturated fat consumed.

Trans-fatty acids or trans fat can also raise the risk of heart disease. Trans fat is formed when liquid vegetable oils go through a chemical process called hydrogenation, which makes the oils into solid fat, like shortening and hard margarine. This process increases the shelf life of foods, including the potato chips, cookies, and fried food that we consume every day. Trans fat behaves like saturated fat, clogging arteries and increasing LDL-C (bad cholesterol) levels.

Take a Clove of Garlic Every Day

Studies show that garlic lowers cholesterol and thins the blood, which may help prevent high blood pressure, heart disease, and stroke.

In laboratory studies, garlic appears to block the growth of cancer cells. Population studies show that people who eat lots of garlic have fewer stomach and colon cancers than those who eat the least. In addition, research has shown that garlic can help boost immunity and reduce high blood sugar levels.

Trans fat may also reduce HDL (good cholesterol levels). The health risks posed by this dangerous fat have prompted many regulatory agencies to require that food manufacturers list trans fat amounts on all nutritional labels. So, when eating packaged foods, try to pick foods labelled 0 g trans fat per serving.

All USANA's macro-optimizers have been analysed and don't contain trans fat. They are delicious, healthy sources of low-glycaemic complex carbohydrates, complete proteins, and beneficial fats in the right ratio. The macro-optimizer drinks and bars are easy to take with you, providing a convenient way to maintain a healthy body with a busy lifestyle.

Nutritional Medicine

Nutritional medicine is unknown to most physicians as well as the public. The benefits of a good exercise program and a healthy diet are well known. Few, however, especially physicians, have any knowledge of the health benefits of taking high-quality nutritional supplements.

Vitamins are a hot issue within the medical field. But the verdict is in. What your doctor doesn't know about nutritional medicine may be killing you. Only about 6 per cent of the graduating physicians in America have received any training in nutrition.

Doctors believe that you don't need supplements and that you get all the nutrients you need from a good diet. Doctor and patients alike must take a long hard look at how they approach healthcare today.

Numerous studies prove that a healthy diet, a good exercise program, and high-quality nutritional supplements are the absolute best way to maintain your health and to regain your health after you have lost it. There are records of amazing results by practising nutritional medicine and patients with multiple sclerosis who have gone from wheelchair-bound to walking again.

Some cancer patients have gone into remission; patients with macular degeneration have found significant visual improvement, and fibromyalgia patients have regained their lives.

Oxidative stress is the underlying cause of all chronic degenerative diseases, like coronary heart disease, stroke, cancer, arthritis, multiple sclerosis, Alzheimer's, and macular degeneration.

Heart disease is not caused by high cholesterol but the inflammation of blood vessels, which can be reduced and even totally eliminated by taking nutritional supplements.

Antioxidants and their supporting nutrients have become our new weapon in the war against our number 1 killer: heart disease. Fruits and vegetables contain thousands of extremely potent bioflavonoids. They also have some anti-allergic and anti-inflammatory properties.

Red wine and grape juice contain polyphenols, which has been proven to reduce the formation of oxidized LDL cholesterol. Grapeseed extract is known as the best antioxidant to prevent chronic inflammatory disease.

Vitamin E is the best antioxidant for the cell wall, vitamin C for the plasma, and glutathione is the best intracellular antioxidant.

All these antioxidants need the so-called antioxidant minerals and B-cofactors to do their job. These ingredients work together in synergy as they accomplish the ultimate goal of defeating oxidative stress.

Doctors are content to let the pharmaceutical companies determine new therapies when they develop new drugs. But our natural antioxidant and immune system are the best defence against the development of chronic degenerative diseases.

There is some good news, however. Medical research is beginning to support the idea of supplementation with a mixture of antioxidants and supporting nutrients.

This mix can enhance traditional chemo and radiation therapy and at the same time protect normal cells from toxic effects. But you don't have to be a physician to start practising nutritional medicine. You as a patient can become proactive about preserving the health you have.

Cellular Nutrition

Cellular nutrition has become more important in our modern society than ever before. Our bodies must face daily an overproduction of free radicals caused by our polluted environment, stressful lifestyles, and malnutrition. However, we can reduce the production of free radicals by avoiding smoking and toxic chemicals and decreasing our stress levels. But most of our bodies are still unable to fight the overwhelming daily attack on our natural defence system.

Balance is the key. If there are not enough antioxidants available to neutralize the free radicals, oxidative stress develops.

Over the past fifty years, nutritional medicine has been concentrating on supplying a nutritional deficiency. Many hours and dollars have been spent trying to determine exactly which nutrients our bodies are depleted of.

Blood and urine tests, hair samples, muscle testing, and more have been conducted in an attempt to determine which nutrients we need to supplement. However, we have been aiming at the wrong target. The problem is not a nutritional deficiency but rather underlying oxidative stress.

Oxidative stress has shown to be the root cause of over seventy degenerative diseases, like heart disease, stroke, cancer, diabetes, arthritis, Alzheimer's disease, dementia, lupus, MS, and the list goes on!

Because the problem is oxidative stress rather than specific nutritional deficiencies, the best approach to prevent or to control oxidative stress is to strengthen our natural defence system through cellular nutrition.

Cellular nutrition means supplying the cells with all nutrients at optimal levels without having to worry about determining which nutrients the cell is deficient in. By providing all the important nutrients at optimal levels, which has been shown to provide a health benefit in the medical literature, we correct automatically any nutritional deficiencies over the next few months.

Cellular nutrition is defined as providing all the nutrients to the cell at optimal levels or to those levels that provide a health benefit according to medical literature. All the antioxidants, along with the supporting B vitamins and minerals, should be at optimal levels.

This is 'preventive medicine' at its best because we can attack the disease process at the core by preventing oxidative stress. Your life and health depend on it. They are far more superior to any drugs your doctor prescribes.

The connection between good nutrition and long-term health is beyond dispute and backed by a wealth of scientific evidence. What we eat and how we eat affect our health on the long term.

Our diet fails in supplying the essential nutrients we need for optimum health. We have put good nutrition on the back burner, and as a result, our diet fails to provide even the minimum levels of nutrients that we need for long-term health.

Only 9 per cent of people consume the five daily servings of fresh fruit and vegetables recommended by the National Cancer Institute that is required each day for optimal health. We are not even getting the minimum of RDA levels of vitamins, minerals, and antioxidants. The RDA levels were designed in the early 1920s and 1930s as minimum requirements of *ten* essential nutrients to protect against acute deficiency diseases, like scurvy (deficiency in vitamin C), rickets (deficiency in vitamin D), and pellagra (deficiency of niacin).The RDA did a good job to eliminate scurvy and rickets, but consuming the RDAs will not even come close to helping prevent a degenerative disease, and our *epidemic* health stats prove that.

The glycaemic index (GI) is a scale from 1 to 100 that measures how quickly carbohydrate foods are broken down into glucose. The original purpose for the glycaemic index was to help diabetics keep their blood sugar under control. The glycaemic index has recently attracted a lot of attention in the bodybuilding, fitness, and weight loss world and has even become the central theme in numerous bestselling diet books as a method to choose the foods that are best for losing weight.

According to advocates of the glycaemic index system, foods that are high on the GI scale such as rice cakes, carrots, potatoes, watermelon, or grape juice are 'unfavourable' and should be avoided because high GI foods are absorbed quickly, raise blood sugar rapidly, and are therefore more likely to convert to fat or cause health problems.

Our modern lifestyle is characterized by degenerative diseases, like stroke, cancer, heart disease, diabetes, arthritis, etc. 96 per cent of the US population dies of a degenerative disease, and over 65 per cent of American adults are overweight or obese (20 per cent to 25 per cent of children).

Most people simply accept the onset of arthritis, heart disease, and diabetes as inevitable results of the ageing process. The truth is, these conditions are largely preventable.

The cause of all this is the build-up of free radicals, which are caused by smoking, stress, lack of exercise, bad nutrition, pollution in air and water, radiation from the sun, and soil depletion.

To combat these free radicals, our body needs a large intake of antioxidants. If there are not enough antioxidants available to neutralize the free radicals, 'oxidative stress' will occur. It's a process by which the oxygen our body uses causes the body to rust like metal does. It's the cause of all degenerative diseases and even the ageing process.

We can get antioxidants out of fruits, vegetables, and nuts. However, it is unpractical and almost impossible to get the required amounts of antioxidants out of our diet alone. The nutritional value of our fruits and vegetables has enormously declined in the past fifty years, caused by soil depletion.

Until the 1940s, farmers used to practice crop rotation and returned essential nutrients back into the soil by mulching, manuring, and churning. Because of growing population and industrialization, it was no longer possible to grow crops that way. So the farmers use large farms and make use of artificial fertilizers. But crops can't make their natural insect repellents with artificial fertilizers, so the farmer has to use chemical pesticides, which are sprayed on the crop and fruits and when we consume those fruits and vegetables. Those chemical pesticides accumulate in our body and cause diseases.

Most of us today are suffering from certain dangerous diet deficiencies, which cannot be remedied until the depleted soils from which our food come are brought into proper mineral balance.

The alarming fact is that fruits and vegetables, now being raised on millions of acres of land that no longer contain enough of certain minerals, are starving us, no matter how much we eat.

In other words, we cannot get the necessary nutrients out of our food. So, in order to get a sufficient number of antioxidants, we have to supplement our diet with high-quality nutritional supplements. It has been scientifically proven that there are substantial health benefits in taking nutritional supplements. Additionally, hundreds of scientific studies have proven that nutritional supplements can significantly reduce the risk of degenerative diseases, and the American Medical Association (AMA) now encourages all adults to supplement daily with a multiple vitamin.

Based on a landmark review of thirty-eight years of scientific evidence by Harvard researchers Dr Robert Fletcher and Dr

Kathleen Fairfield, the conservative *Journal of the American Medical Association (JAMA)* has rewritten its policy guidelines regarding the use of vitamin supplements.

In a striking departure from its previous anti-vitamin rhetoric, *JAMA* (19 June 2002) now recommends that given our nutrient-poor modern diet, supplementation each day with a multiple vitamin is a prudent preventive measure against chronic disease.

The *JAMA* declaration also highlights a growing concern among nutrition experts that the current recommended intakes for vitamins and minerals are too low.

Dr Robert Fletcher, co-author of the groundbreaking *JAMA* studies, states, 'All of us grew up believing that if we ate a reasonable diet, that would take care of our vitamin needs. But the new evidence, much of it in the last couple of years, is that vitamins also prevent the usual diseases we deal with every day—heart disease, cancer, osteoporosis, and birth defects.'

While science and technology have increased our lifespan dramatically over the past few centuries, they have failed to secure for us the holy grail of long-term health. Using the words of Dr Myron Wentz, founder of USANA Health Sciences, 'We are living too short and dying too long.'

4. Good Nutrition as Part of a Healthy Lifestyle

It's a sad fact that about one-third of American adults are overweight. But people can change that by adopting a lifestyle with the right diet. It's important to know how fat is deposited in the body so that you understand how to make the body lose it. Your body needs food to obtain the necessary energy to function and feed its cells. The calories in food have energy, commonly referred to as calories. The more calories food contains, the more fuel the body can get from it.

In order to use the energy from the food, your body has to digest the food first. The process of digestion causes the body to burn some old energy to get the new energy from the food. More energy/calories are burned if it's more difficult to digest the food. The body's fuel is categorized as protein, carbohydrates, or fats. This fuel nourishes the body and keeps the body functioning. The leftover calories are eventually stored in the fat cells. Your body uses a part of the food's fuel for nutrition. The excess fuel is eventually stored up as fat in the 'fat cells' of your body, around the kidneys and liver.

Fat cells are often deposited in the chest, hips, and waist region. As the cells become bigger, your physique acquires a doughy look. The body has a limited number of fat cells, and there is only so much fat these cells can store. Once the threshold is reached, fat begins to accumulate in the muscle lining of your arms and thighs, creating unsightly, flabby limbs.

Eat fat-burning foods. All foods can create fat, but certain foods can actually help burn fat. Some foods have minerals or vitamins that raise metabolism and act as virtual fat burners. There are negative-calorie foods with low calories that burn extra calories during digestion. Other foods, even if you eat them in small quantities, give you a feeling of fullness. They contain very little calories. You will significantly reduce the fat profile of your body if you consume the right whole foods. By eating these fat-burning foods at the right time, in the correct amount, the body fat profile starts to reduce. Add in foods that lower the likelihood of fat depositing in your body for an extra boost.

Here is a list of everyday foods that double as secret fat burners: poultry, salmon, tuna, citrus fruits, apples, berries, oatmeal, vegetables, beans, eggs, almonds and walnuts, and pine nuts.

Add Fat Boosters to Your Diet

This includes mustard, onions, coconut oil, hot peppers, and green tea.

Increase Water Intake

Help your body to reduce fat deposits by drinking more water. The kidneys do not function correctly without enough water intake. If they don't work properly, some of the load is discarded to the liver. If the liver is doing the kidney's work, it can't concentrate on its main job of metabolizing fat. More fat will remain in the body, and fat burning stops. So drinking the right amount of water improves metabolism and keeps your fat burning at full capacity. Water also flushes out toxins and improves the body's ability to stay healthy.

Build Muscles

Muscles keep your metabolism active and help in burning calories. Adding muscle improves your body's fat composition ratio. Because muscles are an active tissue that continually renews itself, it always needs calories. While normal cardio burns fat only during the exercise, weight training builds muscle to ensure that body fat continues to burn throughout the day. The main source of energy for muscles is fat. So even when relaxing or sleeping, you continue to burn calories. The more muscle mass on your frame, the more positive effect on your metabolism. It's important to do weight resistance exercises to build muscle and to avoid your metabolism from getting sluggish and packing on fat.

Now you have the secrets to a beautiful, toned body in the palm of your hands. The only thing standing in the way of a lean, sexy physique is you. Adopt these fat-burning secrets into your lifestyle, and you will see results in a matter of weeks. The right diet plan will show you how to combine the fat-burning foods to keep your body melting away the flab.

There are countless delicious recipes to make the switch painless. Add a weightlifting exercise regime, and you will sculpt your body into an object of desire. The new you is ready to emerge.

5. Preventive Medicine

In the thirteenth century, the philosopher Roger Bacon (c. 1214–1294) believed that the secret to a long and healthy life was depending on the following: exercise, good hygiene, inhaling the breath of a young virgin, a healthy diet, and proper rest. To be able to live to the age of eighty in the thirteenth century was quite an impressive achievement when you consider that there was poor sanitation, there were no antibiotics, and there was no medical care.

Going up in time to the year 2004, the prestigious *Journal of the American Medical Association (JAMA)* published a large study that showed healthy seventy- to ninety-year-old people who adopted the Mediterranean diet, used alcohol in moderation, took physical activity and a non-smoking lifestyle had a 50 per cent decrease in the rate of death. These results are not far off from what Roger Bacon stated more than seven hundred years earlier, with the exception, of course, of inhaling the breath of a young virgin.

These days, research has included some more factors that showed to increase your changes of living a long life. These include good genetics. People whose parents lived to an old age should have more chance of also living a long life. The specific genes involved in the human ageing process are still unknown.

Increased Lipoprotein Size and Increased HDL Cholesterol Levels in Your Blood

There is some evidence that components of your cholesterol may be protective factors for heart disease and stroke, usually seen by people who live to be one hundred. Being lucky! Not being in the wrong place at the wrong time. We all know of people who have been in a bad car accident or were the victim of a violent crime. Others have rare and unexplained illnesses.

Proper Preventive Medical Care

What is preventive medicine? Taking proper steps to avoid the development of illnesses is important, also the early diagnosis of illness. That is why prevention can take several forms. It can involve removing one or more risk factors that can lead to the development of a disease. To quit smoking, for example, may help in preventing a heart attack or stroke. Try to identify a disease at an early stage before it gets to a serious illness or death. For example, a colonoscopy attempts to identify and remove small polyps in the colon before they turn into colon cancer. Keep a close watch on people who have already an illness. Women who have had breast cancer in the past have a much higher risk to develop further breast cancer and will need closer monitoring.

Does proper preventive screening for an elderly patient exist? There are no clear guidelines for the proper screening of an elderly person. Part of the confusion is that there are so many variables among the elderly. Many of the medical specialty societies don't agree as to which tests are suitable to order for elderly patients. This is another problem.

Is a yearly physical exam useful? We are used to the idea that a physical exam every year is an essential factor to assure that we stay healthy.

There are different ideas of what should be included in this exam. Most doctors believe that it should involve a full discussion of all healthcare issues, a full head-to-toe examination, and lab work. The truth is that it has not been proven that this standard format has any benefit for detecting new, potentially life-threatening diseases. It is, however, an opportunity to discuss exercises and to make sure the patient is up to date on his or her immunizations and cancer screening.

Research has shown that yearly ordered test in otherwise healthy seniors are often not beneficial. These tests include chest x-ray, complete blood cell count (CBC), and blood chemistry panel electrocardiogram (EKG).

On the surface, these tests seem to be useful. But in practice, ordering these tests as a routine each year will rarely identify any new diseases.

6. Eat the Right Nutrients When Ageing

When we age, we have to eat well and adjust our eating habits. As we get older, our needs for certain nutrients will change significantly. We produce less saliva, and our swallowing reflexes slow down. As a result, food may not be as easy to digest and to swallow. Many of us experience changes in taste and appetite as we get older, so we may eat less. We also have less stomach acid. That means we don't digest foods or absorb some nutrients as well as we used to.

An Israeli study that looked at 414 elderly patients in hospitals found that less than 20 per cent were well-nourished. The study also found that those with poor dietary habits had less successful outcomes from their visit to the hospital. But even with this information and other studies available, doctors don't always think to check for nutritional deficiencies in older adults.

This is unfortunately because a simple lack of nutrients can easy be mistaken for a more serious illness. Nutritional deficiencies in older people can even be misdiagnosed as dementia.

Vitamin B12 is essential for maintaining healthy blood and nerve function. It's also one of the nutrients that require adequate amounts of stomach secretions to be absorbed. When acid levels decline, getting enough vitamin B12 can be a problem. This is of particular concern for people who use antacids. You can get plenty of vitamin B12 from meats and other animal foods. Clams are the best source of vitamin B12. One small, steamed clam provides an astonishing 9 micrograms of vitamin B12, more than 100 per cent of the DV.

Apart from vitamin B12 deficiency, many people in their late fifties and older may be deficient in vitamin B6. Chickpeas and potatoes are good sources of vitamin B6. One cup of chickpeas contains 1.1 milligrams, slightly more than half of the DV. A baked potato provides 0.6 milligram, or about one-third of the DV.

Another B vitamin that's important for protecting the cardiovascular and nervous systems is folate, which is found in green vegetables, beans, and whole grains. A cup of canned pinto beans, for example, provides 144 milligrams of folate, or more than 33 per cent of the DV. Asparagus is also a good source of folate. One cup of cooked asparagus contains 263 milligrams of folate.

As your bones get older, it's essential to get extra calcium and vitamin D to prevent them from becoming brittle. Many older people think that they can't eat dairy foods because they are 'lactose tolerant', but in fact, most people can eat moderate amounts of dairy without trouble. Low-fat and fat-free (skim) milk, cheese, and yogurt are your best sources of calcium. One cup of fat-free yogurt contains 415 milligrams of calcium, or 41 per cent of the DV. One glass of fat-free milk provides 302 milligrams or 30 per cent of the DV.

Iron is one of several minerals that can be hard to get in the correct amount. Some people don't get enough, while others get too much. Women's need for iron declines in their later years after they stop menstruating.

To ensure that you're getting the right amount of nutrients for your particular needs, it's best to talk to your doctor to find out whether or not you need to take supplements of certain nutrients, such as iron, calcium, vitamin D, and vitamin B12.

Even though we may need to eat more of certain foods in order to live longer, researchers are finding that the opposite can also be true: people who eat less may live more years.

A Louisiana State University study followed forty-eight people for six months as they either followed a normal diet or different types of calorie-restricted diets. It found that prolonged calorie restriction can lower people's fasting insulin levels and their body temperature, which are both markers of longevity.

Experts think that calorie restriction 'resets' your metabolism so it works more efficiently, and your body shifts its focus from growth and reproduction to long-term survival. And when you take less calories, your body produces less free radicals as it turns food into energy.

However, it's hard for humans to reap the benefits from calorie reduction that lab animals have shown. For those among us who like to eat, it's probably not a viable strategy. In addition, drastically reducing your calories without medical supervision can leave you malnourished.

For now, a good way to get some benefit from calorie reduction is to make sure that you eat a 'prudent' diet that provides the nutrients you need without excessive calories. If you do decide to restrict your calories, talk to your doctor to make sure your diet meets your nutritional needs. See also my article about flavonoids.

Chapter 2

7. Healthy for Life with Natural Digestive Enzymes

To be healthy for life, it is important to consume eight to ten servings of fruit and vegetables daily, and many of these should be raw that we consider to be 'life food' because they contain those natural digestive enzymes. I also recommend that your diet is free from high-glycaemic carbohydrates and sugar.

Because you will not be spiking your blood sugar, this will also keep your yeast in check and is the answer if you have problems with recurrent yeast infections.

It will keep your blood sugar lower, which is also critical to keep a balanced GI flora. I also advise you to consume more good fat and good protein and reduce the amount of bad fat and bad protein that's in your diet now. So I recommend that you take high-quality, complete, and balanced nutritional supplements at the optimal levels that have been proven to provide a health benefit in medical literature.

However, even if you practice a healthy lifestyle, there can be problems sometimes which are out of your control. Science has shown that when we get older, the production of digestive enzymes becomes less.

When you combine this with a diet of highly processed foods without any natural digestive enzymes, for many of us, this results in having less capacity to digest our micronutrients as we once did.

You could have irritable bowel, GI distress, reflux, and chronic fatigue. I would advise you to consider adding digestive enzymes to your diet and consume one to three high-quality digestive enzymes prior to or with your meal. This will allow you to replenish your digestive enzymes and better digest and absorb the nutrients from your food and supplements.

As a bonus, you will usually notice an improvement in your GI tract and general health within four to six weeks of starting digestive enzymes.

Of course, you adjust the number of enzymes you are consuming based on your response. If you respond well with one digestive tablet prior to or with your meal, then I suggest you stay at this level. You respond better with two to three tablets, then this may be the level you need to take.

I also suggest that you take high-quality probiotics every other day. This will bring your GI flora back into balance and suppress the bad bacteria and yeast. If you have to take a course of antibiotics for an infection, then take a packet of probiotics daily while you are on the antibiotics and for at least two weeks afterwards. This will help you better to avoid many of the terrible GI complications which antibiotics can cause and protect your health by bringing this 'garden within' back into balance as soon as possible.

If you are eating a healthy diet and didn't have to take antibiotics, then you may find that after a few months of taking probiotics, you don't need to continue taking them. However, for many people who have such good health benefits or are concerned with the antibiotics that are in our food supply, which cannot be avoided by most of us, continuing to take probiotics every other day or at least a few times per week is a good idea.

Keeping your 'garden within' into balance with natural digestive enzymes is a key aspect of general health and an optimal immune system.

8. Eating Healthy—the GI Way!

Researchers continue to gather evidence regarding the GI's far-reaching health benefits since the positive effects of a low-GI eating plan were discovered in the 1980s.

Most nutritionists and health professionals agree today that a low-GI diet plan not only helps to keep you slim but also lowers your risk of getting type 2 diabetes, heart disease, and some forms of cancer. The diet has also proved to improve memory, concentration, and mood.

GI means glycaemic index. It is a measure of how long it takes to break your food down into glucose. The key to the low-GI diet is focused on slow-acting carbohydrate foods, which help to keep your blood glucose level steady.

The glycaemic index is a way to rank foods according to the effect they have on our blood glucose levels. This is especially true in regard to carbohydrates.

Specifically, the glycaemic index measures how much a 50-gram portion of carbohydrates raises your blood sugar levels compared with a control. The control is either white bread or pure glucose.

All carbohydrates cause some temporary rise in your blood glucose level. This is called the glycaemic response. And this response is affected by a variety of factors, including the amount of food eaten, the type of carbohydrates, the method used to prepare the food, as well as the degree of processing, to name just a few.

The slower your body processes the food, the slower the insulin is released, and the healthier the overall effect is on your body. And it's the foods that raise your blood sugar level slowly that you, as a person desiring to lose weight, want to eat. And there are several reasons for this.

First, these foods—many of which you'll discover are high in fibre—will just keep you feeling fuller for a longer period or time. And any of you who have been on a diet can be thankful for this.

What affects the GI?

1. level of food processing
2. physical structure, starch, protein, acidity, soluble fibre, and fat

How can low-GI carbs help with weight loss?

1. It delays hunger pangs.
2. It promotes a faster fat loss.
3. It causes less drop in metabolic rate.
4. It reduces dramatic fluctuations in blood glucose levels.
5. It reduces insulin demands significantly.

These are the benefits from low-GI diets.

1. is easy to follow
2. has greater variety of foods
3. supports exercise program
4. benefits blood lipid profile
5. is environmentally friendly

Foods containing sugar are not necessarily high GI. Sucrose (table sugar) has moderate GI.

The basics of a low-GI diet is to eat whole-grain bread, mountain bread, of stoneground bread, pasta, noodles, barley, sweet potato, legumes, oats, muesli, low-GI cereals.

Here are steps to long-term weight management.

1. Diet—eat to appetite with the right foods.
2. Exercise regularly and incorporate more intense sessions.
3. Be active in daily life.
4. Have a good relationship with food (women).

Heart Health

When eating meals that cause blood glucose levels to spike, it tends to lower 'good' HDL cholesterol and raise triglycerides, harmful fats that increase your risk of heart disease.

High blood glucose also produces unstable forms of oxygen molecules, called free radicals, that damage arteries and make cholesterol more likely to stick on artery walls.

The raised levels of insulin, produced to cope with surges of blood glucose, set in motion changes that raise your blood pressure. This makes your blood more likely to form clots and increase inflammation, which doctors know is closely related to heart attack risks.

Cancer Risk

According to the latest research, high blood glucose levels may increase your chances of getting cancer. It seems that the high insulin levels promote an environment in which it is easier for certain tumours to grow. Research is still going on, and it is too early to be absolutely certain about the connection between blood glucose and cancer. Yet there is a reason for concern for the following types of cancer: colon and rectal, breast, endometrial (womb lining), prostate, and pancreatic cancer.

The Road to Diabetes

It has been known since a long time that a diet high with fast-acting, high-GI foods will significantly increase your risk of type 2 diabetes. In type 2 diabetes, your body can't make enough insulin to keep your blood glucose levels under control. Before you reach that stage, your body may develop insulin resistance and/or metabolic syndrome (syndrome X)—a prediabetic state in which your body progressively struggles to control blood glucose.

Many people are unaware that they have these conditions, yet studies show that they are increasingly common in Australia, New Zealand, South Africa, and the UK. More than 10 per cent of adults have insulin resistance. Fortunately, you don't develop diabetes overnight, and the journey towards diabetes can be redirected at any point. Eating more slow-acting foods is one of the best ways of preventing or reversing this condition. The earlier you start, the better.

Mood and Memory

The brain is very sensitive to the levels of glucose in the blood. Both high and low levels can cause problems with your mood and memory. Low levels may cause symptoms of depression, poor memory, and low concentration, while high levels of blood glucose also impair the brain, shrinking the part that stores memories and increasing the risk of dementia.

The answer is to keep your blood glucose levels steady by eating a low-GI diet.

To follow this diet is simple. There is no need of counting calories, no food is forbidden, and because the way you are eating, you are unlikely to feel hungry.

Focus on eating a low-GI meal, although eating a medium-GI meal now and then will do your diet no harm.

This is not meant to be a strict dietary regime that is endured for a few weeks and dropped but a healthy eating plan for life. So, choose the meals that entice you.

Here, follow these ten tips to lower the GI of your diet.

The following are practical tips to help you make the change to low-GI eating. There is no specific order. Basically, you should attack the changes that you think you'll find easiest first. Make the changes gradually—it can take six weeks for a new behaviour to become a habit.

1. Aim to eat seven servings of fruits and vegetables every day, preferably of three or more different colours. Make sure you fill half your dinner plate with vegetables.
2. Cut back on potatoes. Have one or two boiled new potatoes, or make a cannellini bean and potato mash, replacing half the potato with cannellini beans. Try other lower-GI starchy vegetables for a change, like a piece of sweet potato.
3. Choose a real grainy bread, such as stoneground whole meal, real sourdough bread, or a soy and linseed bread. (Look for the GI symbol on the breads when you buy.)
4. Start the day with smart carbs, like natural muesli or traditional (not instant) porridge oats, or one of the lower-GI processed breakfast cereals that will trickle fuel into your engine.

5. Look for the lower-GI rice (basmati, Doongara, Clever rice, or Moolgiri), and choose low-GI whole grains such as pearl barley, buckwheat, burghul (bulgul), or quinoa.

6. Learn to love legumes and eat them often. Add red kidney beans to a chili, chickpeas to a stir-fry, a four-bean salad to a barbecue, and beans or lentils to a casserole or soup.

7. Include at least one low-GI carb food at every meal and choose low-GI snacks.

8. Incorporate a lean protein source with every meal, such as lean meat, skinless chicken, eggs, fish and seafood, or legumes and tofu if you are vegetarian.

9. Use the GI-lowering effect or acidic foods like vinegar, citrus fruit, and sourdough. Add vinaigrette dressing to salads and sprinkle lemon juice on vegetables like asparagus. Acids slow down the digestion of carbs and lower the overall GI of the meal.

10. Limit (preferably avoid) high-GI refined flour products, whether from the supermarket or home-baked, such as biscuits, cakes, pastries, crumpets, crackers, and biscuits.

As a general rule of thumb, the less processed a food is, the lower its GI value.

The more work the body must do in digesting it, that means the slower the sugar is released, and that is good news for keeping blood glucose levels steady.

After a few weeks of eating the GI way, you'll wonder why you didn't start sooner as you may feel more energetic. And if the nutritionists are correct, adopting the low-GI eating plan may be the best thing you've ever done for your health.

9. Vitamin D Deficiency

Do you get enough vitamin D in your day?

Around 90 per cent of your vitamin D is produced by your skin; only 10 per cent comes from food. The UVB rays that make vitamin D are around most of the day in summer, but only around noon in winter.

From a large Australian study (AusDiab), 58 per cent of females and 35 per cent of males have low levels of vitamin D in winter–springtime. Low levels of vitamin D can cause osteoporosis, which increases the risk of fractures in older people, multiple sclerosis, rheumatoid arthritis, muscle weakness, memory loss, and some cancers.

USANA's vitamin D3 supplement (cholecalciferol) provides the same form of vitamin as we make in the skin. Supplements are a reasonable way to improve vitamin D status if more sun exposure is not practical.

10. Synergy in Vitamin and Mineral Supplementation

Most people who take vitamin and mineral supplements self-prescribe to what they think they should take, not even what is fashionable. As well as being a waste of money, this is likely to do more harm than good.

Why? Because taking an extra dose of one vitamin can lower levels of another. Falling short of a particular mineral can prevent the absorption of another seemingly unrelated one. A dose of an isolated vitamin or mineral that is too high can produce the same symptoms as a deficiency of another nutrient. This is what nutritionists call synergy, and it explains why taking extra calcium to build stronger bones may backfire on you. Too much calcium in the body can cause a deficiency in iron, zinc, magnesium, and phosphorous by preventing their proper absorption. All these minerals are vital for good bone health, and their ongoing deficiency can lead to osteoporosis—the condition you were trying to prevent by taking calcium supplements.

Vitamin D, which is also known as the sunshine vitamin since the body needs exposure to sunlight to make it, enhances the absorption of calcium, but too much can cause a potassium deficiency.

Vitamin A is an antioxidant that is said to help to prevent premature ageing. It does help to maintain the surfaces of the body, including the skin, but too much increases the body's need for another antioxidant, vitamin E, which protect against heart disease.

Vitamin C remains the most popular of the self-prescribed supplements: an estimated ten million Britons take it every day. Research papers now prove that it has powerful antioxidant properties that protect against cancer and heart disease and show how it boosts the immune system to protect against infections and can even speed up wound healing. Yet not many people know that it works much better in the presence of vitamin A or that to use it properly, the body needs calcium.

Ask any alternative cancer specialists what nutrients their patients should be eating, and they will specify bioflavonoids. Though not a true vitamin, these are a group of biologically active substances found in plants that are sometimes called vitamin P.

As well as cancer-fighting properties, they also have an antibacterial effect in the body, where they promote healthy circulation, stimulate bile production for the breakdown of fats, and lower blood cholesterol levels.

Foods that are rich in flavonoids include apples, beetroot, blackberries, cabbage, carrots, cauliflower, cherries, dandelions, lentils, lettuce, oranges, parsley, plums, peas, potatoes, rhubarb, rose hips, spinach, tomatoes, walnuts, and watercress. But what you may not know is that they all work even better when taken with vitamin C, and vice versa.

Synergistic partners are rarely monogamous. To correct a deficiency in vitamin A, you also need six additional nutrients: choline; zinc; vitamins C, D, and E; plus the essential fatty acids found in oily fish or evening primrose oil supplements.

To restore normal levels of vitamin C, you need the bioflavonoids, vitamin A, plus calcium and magnesium. Those last two minerals are so closely linked that if you plan to take a supplement, you need to follow a ratio of 2:1 in favour of the calcium. So, if you are taking 800 milligrams of calcium, you need to take 400 milligrams of magnesium too. To correct a shortage of calcium in the hope of building stronger bones, you also need magnesium; boron; manganese; phosphorous; vitamins A, C, D, and F; plus essential fatty acids. To complicate the picture further, synergy may not affect the whole body but only specific cells, so the impact of what you are doing may be hidden. Smoking, for example, wipes out vitamin C in the body, but this deficiency may be confined to the cells of the lungs.

As you can see, when taking supplements, you have to make sure that the vitamin and mineral balance in your body is maintained.

11. A Healthy Brain Diet Prevents Stroke

Research has shown that when people are missing certain nutrients, their mental performance drops. When people meet their nutritional needs, they are okay. But even if they are not getting enough water, their mind can get fuzzy. The thirst mechanism slows down when we age.

Your brain needs vitamin B.

The most essential nutrients to keep your mind sharp are probably the vitamin B complex. Your body needs the B vitamins for the transformation of food into mental energy and for the manufacturing and repairing of brain tissue. 'Thiamine, niacin, and vitamin B6 and B12 deficiencies can all cause malfunction of the brain,' says Vernon Mark, MD, author of *Reversing Memory Loss*. 'In fact, pellagra, a niacin deficiency, used to be the main cause of admissions into mental hospitals,' he explains. Research has shown that when children are given 5 milligrams thiamine instead of the daily value of 1.5 milligrams, they achieve remarkably higher scores when they are given tests of mental functioning, Dr Mark adds.

Nowadays, many cereals, breads, and pastas are enriched with thiamine and niacin so that most people are getting enough of these vitamins. Niacin deficiencies have become extremely rare, especially in this country. But in older people or those who frequently drink alcohol, levels of thiamine can drop low enough to cause memory problems, says Dr Mark.

The best way to make sure you get enough brain-boosting B vitamins is to eat foods that contain enriched grains. One cup of enriched spaghetti, for example, has 0.3 milligram of thiamine, or 20 per cent of the daily value (DV), and 2 milligrams of niacin, or 10 per cent of the DV. Meat is also a good source for getting these nutrients. Three ounces of pork tenderloin, for example, provides 0.8 milligram of thiamine, 53 per cent of the DV, while 3 ounces of chicken breast delivers 12 milligrams or 60 per cent of the DV for niacin.

It's not so easy when we get older to get extra amounts of vitamin B6 and B12 because it's harder for the body to absorb them. After the age of fifty-five, it's common to be low in these vitamins because the lining of the stomach is changing. When you get older, it's a good idea to get more than the DV of both of these nutrients. Vitamin B6 is abundant in baked potatoes, bananas, chickpeas, and turkey. One baked potato provides 0.4 milligram of vitamin B6, 20 per cent of the DV, and one banana provides 0.7 milligram or 35 per cent of the DV. For vitamin B12, meat and shellfish are good choices.

Maintaining Blood Flow to the Brain

There should be sufficient blood flow to the brain in order to avoid memory problems.

When adequate blood flow is not maintained, the brain and memory begin to perform poorly. The lack of blood to the brain is often caused by a build-up of cholesterol and fat in the arteries, the same problem that leads to heart disease and stroke. This condition is not only preventable through diet, but it is even at least partially reversible. The primary cause of cardiovascular disease—clogged arteries in the heart and the brain—is too much saturated fat in the diet. Keep your intake of saturated fat low by cooking with small amounts of liquid oils, such as olive or canola oil instead of margarine or butter, and by minimizing your intake of fatty foods, such as full-fat mayonnaise, rich desserts, and fatty meats.

It's also important to get plenty of fruits and vegetables. Fruits and vegetables are packed with antioxidants, compounds that block the effects of harmful oxygen molecules called free radicals. This is important because when free radicals damage the harmful low-density-lipoprotein (LDL) cholesterol, it becomes stickier and more likely to stick to artery walls.

Studies have proven that antioxidants in fruits and vegetables can help prevent Alzheimer's disease. In 2002, researchers studied nearly

5,500 people and found that those who ate diets rich in antioxidants, vitamin C and E, lowered their risk of developing Alzheimer's disease. Citrus fruits, kiwi fruit, sprouts, broccoli, and cabbage are packed with vitamin C. While whole grains, nuts, milk, and egg yolks contain vitamin E.

The combination of eating plenty of fruits and vegetables and reducing fat in your diet will help to keep your arteries clear, including those leading to your brain. Actually, it can help restore blood flow through your arteries that have already started to close up.

Coffee can improve memory function. It's not without reason that millions of Americans jump-start their day with steaming cups of coffee. The caffeine in coffee has been shown to improve mental functioning, including memory.

In one study, Dutch researchers used a chemical to block short-term memory in sixteen healthy people. They found that giving these people 250 milligrams of caffeine—about the amount of three cups of coffee—quickly restored their powers of recall. However, too much coffee can be bad, if only the java buzz wears off within six to eight hours. For some people, at least, the after-coffee slump can result in mental fogginess.

Everyone has different reactions to caffeine. For people who rarely drink coffee, having a cup or two can definitely improve performance and memory. But if you drink coffee throughout the day, you quickly build up tolerance, and you won't get the same benefits. In fact, too much caffeine can make you nervous and reduce your concentration.

Don't kill your brain cells. 'Killing brain cells is not the best way to get a high score in the memory department. Yet that's exactly what many of us do to our grey matter. Drinking too much alcohol can cause a significant decrease in memory function.' In fact, even small amounts of alcohol can damage cells in the brain responsible for memory.

Many doctors recommend stopping drinking alcohol all together to keep your mind at its sharpest. At the very least, it's a good idea to limit yourself to one or two drinks—meaning 12 ounces of beer, 5 ounces of wine or 11/2 ounces of liquor—a day. When you do drink, choose red wine. It contains resveratrol, a compound that may keep your brain young.

Optimal Diet for Your Brain

You can't prevent Alzheimer's disease and dementia altogether, but you can keep them at bay longer with a heart-healthy diet that focuses on the nutrients that have been found to be critical for brain function and ageing.

Aim for a body mass index of 23 to 25. Being overweight increases your risk for diabetes, metabolic syndrome, and hypertension, which leads to vascular disease and brain damage.

Choose Dairy

Eat one serving of low-fat, low-sugar dairy once a day, such as milk, plain yogurt, cottage cheese, or ricotta cheese.

Epidemiology studies show that people who drink milk are less likely to develop Alzheimer's disease.

Toast to a Young Brain

Drink one glass of red wine or 4 ounces of purple grape juice or pomegranate juice a day. They contain resveratrol, a compound that doctors believe activates a gene that is associated with longevity.

Eat Berries

When you eat one cup of berries a day, it gives your brain resveratrol and other flavonoids that strengthen your resistance against the development of chronic diseases associated with ageing.

Drink Some Juice

Drink 8 ounces of fruit juice high in vitamin C daily. Three times a week, substitute a glass of vegetable juice that you buy or make on your own for the fruit juice. Antioxidants and other compounds in those juices help protect the brain from dementia.

Include Fish Oil in Your Diet

Omega-3 fatty acids are powerful agents for a healthy heart and arteries. When you eat oily cold water fish such as sardines or mackerel, you will ensure that you get enough omega-3. You can also substitute with 2,000 to 3,000 milligrams of fish oil or flaxseed oil per day. Walnuts are also rich in omega-3. Eating eight to ten walnuts per day or using walnut oil in your salads of dark-green vegetables will help protect your brain.

Drink Green Tea Every Day

Green tea is rich in antioxidants and has proved to reduce the risk of dementia. Experts recommend drinking one to two cups a day.

Use Multivitamins

To include those in your diet is particularly important for older, inactive adults whose calorie intake doesn't supply the micronutrients that they need. Choose a multivitamin without iron or reduced iron if you are not anaemic or menstruating.

Consider Vitamin D Supplements

Vitamin D is a new shining start in the role of brain development and function, and many people are deficient without knowing it. We get about 95 per cent of our vitamin D from sunlight, but young people who work long hours and elderly adults who are homebound often don't get enough sunlight to fill their vitamin D requirements.

Avoid omega-6 fats. The omega-6 fatty acids in corn, safflower, and sesame oils aren't as healthy as omega-3s found in olive and canola oil. So use those oils sparingly.

Nourish Your Brain

An overall brain-healthy diet is low in refined carbohydrates (found in sugars, baked food, candy, and other sweets, for example), red meats, and trans fats. It's high in fatty fish, poultry, soy protein, fruits, vegetables, and legumes.

12. How Food Affects Our Mood—the Right Nutrition to Beat Depression

As we all know, many people seek emotional comfort in food when feeling down. But many people experience just the opposite. Instead of comfort, the food makes them feel worse, listless, moody, and fatigued. Researchers are still uncertain about the connection between food and mood. According to studies, for some individuals, diet can cause depression.

What you eat can lift your mood, but if you eat the wrong food, it can put you down. On the other side, what you don't eat can have as great an impact as what you do eat.

The Food–Mood Factor

About 100 billion nerve cells in our brain, called neurons, control everything we do, from thinking and feeling to taking a walk. Neurons use neurotransmitters in order to communicate with each other. These brain chemicals are called serotonin, dopamine, and norepinephrine.

Apart from communication, these chemicals also can have a significant effect on our mood. For example, if we are in need of serotonin, depression and insomnia and food cravings may result. On the other hand, when serotonin levels are high, we can experience feelings of calm and well-being. When levels of dopamine and norepinephrine in our brain are changed, it can have similar results.

Fish can have a positive effect on our mood. It's for good reason that Charlie the Tuna always looks happy! Tuna and other oily cold-water fish are the best sources of omega-3 fatty acids, which, according to studies, are linked to lower rates of depression.

Omega-3 polyunsaturated fatty acids may be beneficial to good mental health. Experts recommend to have two servings of fish with a high omega-3 content, such as salmon, sardines, and Spanish mackerel. Other sources include canola oil and flaxseed oil.

Recent research has found that omega-3 boosts moods even in non-depressed people. Scientists at the University of Pittsburgh measured the levels of omega-3 in the blood of 106 healthy adults, and after giving them psychological tests, they found that the people with the highest omega-3 levels in their blood scored 49 per cent to 58 per cent better in the test than the people with the lowest omega-3 levels.

Carbohydrates have a calming effect. Diets high in carbohydrate showed a rise in brain concentrations of the amino acid tryptophan.

The tryptophan is converted in our body to serotonin. That may be the reason why, for many people, comfort foods that are high in carbohydrates can lower feelings of depression. For others who don't eat as many carbohydrates, they may feel grouchy and depressed.

Some people, of course, can eat loads of pasta, potatoes, and bread without noticing any difference. But for others, known by scientists as carbohydrate cravers, the effects can be quite significant. It could be that carbohydrate cravings are the result of the body's attempt to counteract low serotonin levels. Many people who eat spaghetti with marinara sauce and French bread for lunch get sleepy because that carbohydrate-rich meal raises their serotonin levels.

Controlling Mood Swings

It's a well-known fact that some people experience mood swings at certain times. For some women, it's just before their menstrual periods. And some people, they now found out, can improve their moods during low times by eating more carbohydrates.

At a research conducted at Harvard University, women suffering from premenstrual mood swings were asked to drink about 7 1/2 ounces of a specially formulated high-carbohydrate drink once a month, just before their periods. Within hours of having the drink, they experience significant reductions in depression, anger, and confusion, the researchers found.

You can get a similar amount of carbohydrate like the women in the study by eating a small portion of a high-carbohydrate food, like a cup of whole-wheat pasta, some baked potatoes, or a half cup of raisins.

When feeling depressed, you probably know from experience that droopy, let-down feeling that sometimes occurs after drinking a large cappuccino or binging on your favourite cookies.

It's a reality. 'Consuming too much sugar or caffeine definitely contributes to feelings of depression for sensitive individuals,' says Dr Christensen. Experts aren't sure sugar gives some people the blues, but it may be related to the amount you consume, says Dr Christensen. While indulging in an occasional candy bar or doughnut can trigger a 'sugar buzz' that temporarily boosts your spirits, a steady diet of sugar seems to be linked with depression.

Dr Christensen and a colleague led a study in which twenty people with serious depression were asked to cut all sugar and caffeine from their diets. After three weeks, these people were significantly less depressed.

Although the effects of caffeine on mood haven't been studied extensively, there's evidence that cutting back on coffee or other high-caffeine drinks, may lift your spirits, especially if you usually drink it a lot.

Doctor's advice is, 'Have a bit of chocolate,' says Jennefer Ramos Galluzzi, PhD, of Housatonic Community College in Bridgeport, Connecticut. 'In small amounts, it's a mood booster.' And who is going to argue with that?

13. The Benefits of a Ketogenic Diet

The ketogenic diet is a new form of dieting where low carbohydrates, adequate protein, and high fats are consumed. The goal of a ketogenic diet is to deplete the body's glycogen reserves so that it relies on fat and protein for energy. The body then undergoes ketosis, which is a metabolic state in which your liver produces a high number of ketones as an alternative fuel source for the brain. This form of dieting is quite popular, with dozens of pictures showing before and after results circulating all over social media.

The following are some benefits of the keto diet and how it may help in achieving your goals.

Weight Loss

Several studies have proven that people on a low-carbohydrate, high-fat diet burn fat at a faster rate than those with a high-carbohydrate, low-fat diet. This is primarily because lower insulin levels caused by the low-carbohydrate diet (keto) help to remove excess water from the body. During ketosis, you feel less hungry, which can be extremely beneficial to control caloric intake and to promote overall weight loss. It has been experienced that low-carb diets are also effective in reducing visceral fat, primarily stored in the abdominal cavity.

Mental Performance

The ketones produced from a low-carbohydrate diet are a much more efficient source of energy than glucose. Studies have indicated that they can improve cognitive impairment and even help with Alzheimer's and Parkinson's diseases. The high-fat diet helps to maintain the balance of essential omega-3s and omega-6s, which are vital for optimal brain function. In addition, ketosis is able to boost mitochondria production and adenosine triphosphate within the brain's memory cells, which results in improving mental performance and clarity.

Reduced Risk of Chronic Disease

A ketogenic diet can boost the body's defence against a variety of conditions. By reducing inflammation and improving mitochondrial function, it can help to reduce the risk of developing several chronic diseases. Cancer cells typically possess abnormal mitochondria, which need an increased supply of glycogen. Ketosis allows to feed the normal cells while starving the cancer cells as they are unable to use the ketones for energy because of their dysfunctional mitochondria.

Blood Pressure Control

High blood pressure significantly increases the risk of several diseases and is a leading cause of deaths worldwide. A low-carbohydrate diet has been proven to be more effective than a low-fat diet in reducing blood pressure. In fact, some claim that it is just as effective as taking pills. This combined with the weight loss derived from a ketogenic diet is sure to vastly improve cardiovascular health and function.

Mental Performance

The ketones produced from a low-carbohydrate diet are a much more efficient source of energy than glucose. Studies have indicated that they can improve cognitive impairment and even help with Alzheimer's and Parkinson's diseases. The high-fat diet helps to maintain the balance of essential omega-3s and omega-6s, which are vital for optimal brain function. In addition, ketosis is able to boost mitochondria production and adenosine triphosphate within the brain's memory cells, which results in improving mental performance and clarity.

Reduced Risk of Chronic Disease

A ketogenic diet can boost the body's defence against a variety of conditions. By reducing inflammation and improving mitochondrial function, it can help to reduce the risk of developing several chronic diseases. Cancer cells typically possess abnormal mitochondria, which need an increased supply of glycogen. Ketosis allows to feed the normal cells while starving the cancer cells as they are unable to use the ketones for energy because of their dysfunctional mitochondria.

Blood Pressure Control

High blood pressure significantly increases the risk of several diseases and is a leading cause of deaths worldwide. A low-carbohydrate diet has been proven to be more effective than a low-fat diet in reducing blood pressure. In fact, some claim that it is just as effective as taking pills. This combined with the weight loss derived from a ketogenic diet is sure to vastly improve cardiovascular health and function.

It has been shown by numerous studies in the realm of nutrition science that this form of dieting can have a very positive impact on your overall health and bodily function. As long as you can find a way to maintain the discipline, the rewards are abundant. For those who have not been able to gain many results from traditional methods, the keto approach is definitely something worth considering.

14. The Benefits of Raw Food

It is a well-known fact that with high temperatures when cooking, some vitamins will be destroyed, particularly vitamin C and vitamin B9 (folic acid). It may also render minerals inorganic and denature some proteins, and it certainly destroys the life force in raw plant food. Cooking kills all enzymes. Their activity increases as the temperature rises, but only up to 42 degrees Celsius, after which enzyme activity slows down. If the food is heated to 48 degrees Celsius for more than half an hour, all enzymes are completely destroyed. In contrast, dry heat would not be destructive to enzymes until around 150 degrees Celsius, but this is theoretical as all foods contain moisture.

Thus, cooking and pasteurization completely destroy the natural, health-giving enzymes that are present in all raw foods.

Like vitamins, enzymes are present in all vegetable and animal tissue in their natural state. They are the biological catalysts that trigger off all the millions of chemical changes that are taking place within the human body, every second of our lives. There are tens of thousands of enzymes working away in our body—with something like 50,000 in the liver alone! And each of them has its own specific purpose.

When food intake is above starvation level and all the necessary nutrients are provided, the less food that is consumed on a long-term basis by humans, animals, and insects, the longer they live. When the air temperature rises, that causes insects to be much more active, but they die sooner because their enzymes are used up more rapidly. Enzyme supply may well be the yardstick of vitality.

It is accepted in general that the enzymes in food cannot work in our bodies, although Dr Edward Howell has written a book, *Food Enzymes for Health and Longevity*, in which he states that there is strong evidence to the contrary.

The enzymes in raw food commence the digestion of each morsel the moment the food's cell walls are ruptured by chewing. The food enzymes assist our own digestive enzymes, easing the load on the organs that produce our enzymes, particularly the pancreas. When humans eat cooked food, the pancreas is enlarged due to overwork.

In fact, Oriental people on a high-carbohydrate cooked diet, mainly rice, have pancreas approximately half as big as Westerners.

All animals in the wild consume abundant enzymes in their always-raw diets. Some have a separate stomach in which the food enzymes predigest food before the body's digestive enzymes are called upon, for example, the rumen in the cow.

The enzyme content of organically grown food that has ripened at its source (on the tree, vine, etc.) is significantly higher than conventionally grown foods.

When raw food enzymes reach the bowel, they encourage the friendly gut bacteria by binding any oxygen present, thus eliminating the aerobic conditions in which harmful bacteria grow and cause putrefaction, toxaemia, and ultimately degenerative diseases, including cancer.

When the harmful bacteria are gone, beneficial bacteria, like acidophilus and bifidobacteria, can flourish and carry out their vital functions, including the manufacture of B vitamins, digestion of fibre, and production of natural 'antibiotics' against pathogenic bacteria.

In the highly cooked Western diet, a high incidence of arthritis, diabetes, heart disease, cancer, and other degenerative conditions is exactly what can be expected as a result of enzyme damage.

In contrast, the remarkable therapeutic value of a short-term diet of raw fresh fruits and vegetables and/or their juices, which have been employed all over the world, is exactly what we would expect.

15. Protein: Why It's Important for Wellness, Fitness, and Weight Management

Protein plays a fundamental role in our overall body health and wellness. It helps with weight control and in building, maintaining, and repairing muscles. Studies have shown that a meal high in protein can help you feel fuller longer, which helps further with weight management. But how much do we really need? It could be more than you think!

The 'average' adult, according to the European Food Safety Authority, needs 0.83 grams of protein per kilogram of body weight. However, this level increases with the level of activity undertaken. Protein dietician Orla Walsh says that active adults and those training should consume between 1.2 grams and 1.5 grams of protein per kilogram of body weight per day depending on the level of intensity of the exercise. It is considered safe to consume up to 1.6 grams of protein per kilogram of body weight per day.

Many people may not know that pregnant women require additional intake of 1 gram, 9 grams, and 28 grams per day for the first, second, and third trimesters, respectively, and breastfeeding women need an additional intake of 19 grams per day during the first six months and 13 grams per day thereafter. Infants, children, and adolescents require between 0.83 grams and 1.31 grams of protein per kilogram of body weight per day depending on age.

If you are a vegetarian or vegan, you may find getting enough protein more of a challenge simply because there are fewer protein sources available and less 'grab and go' availability.

So what does protein *do* for us? At the most basic level, protein is needed for every cell in the body, so to be healthy and well and to have the best possible body, skin, hair, and nails, you must get the correct amount of protein every day. Muscles are made of protein, and protein maintains, repairs, and builds muscle. The more muscle you have, the faster your metabolism goes, and a healthy metabolism is key to lowering body fat and maintaining a healthy body fat percentage, which is beneficial for our health throughout our lives. If you are active, a protein shake or adding protein to a smoothie after activity will help repair muscles and replenish the body. A great choice is that protein 2-in-1 Plant Protein Super Foods as the range also contains not only organic plant protein but also added nutrition like vitamin C for reducing tiredness and fatigue and supporting a healthy immune system.

Don't forget that muscles are not just located externally but also internally, e.g. the heart is a muscle. Our muscles are constantly breaking down and repairing, and they need protein for fuel and repair. Without adequate protein, the body will stop functioning at optimum level, and illness could follow.

So is that all we need to know?

Not quite. Firstly, all proteins are not equal. Some will come with attendant saturated fat (think, e.g. red meat or cheese), and other sources can be highly processed, contain artificial ingredients, or be high in refined sugars.

Secondly, some proteins are not complete proteins. That means they do not contain all the essential amino acids the body needs every day to be healthy and well but can't make itself. These are leucine, isoleucine, lysine, methionine, histidine, phenylalanine, threonine, tryptophan, and valine. As the body can't make these amino acids, we must get them from our food.

Finally, it's not just the amount of protein we need to be aware of but also when we need to consume that amount. The body can only process and utilize so much protein at one sitting, so key to protein consumption is to spread it evenly across the day.

So to make sure you are getting your protein consumption right, why not take this mini protein challenge with five easy steps?

Start in the morning by working out how much protein you need to eat that day based on the above reference intakes, your lifestyle, and your exercise levels.

Write down in a notebook how much protein you actually consume that day.

Consider the kind of protein you are consuming and how that fits with your lifestyle and health priorities, e.g. is it organic? Is it low in saturated fat? Is it free from chemicals and additives? Is it free from refined sugar? Lactose-free? Vegan? You decide!

Be aware of when you are consuming your protein and if you are having it throughout the day. Don't just add up the total amount of protein. It must be taken throughout the day.

Conclude if you are getting your protein intake right or need to make changes.

Consuming the right type and the right amount of protein for your lifestyle and exercise level at the right time will ensure you support your total body health and wellness and help you attain your fitness and weight management goals.

16. How to Increase Testosterone Levels

High-fat diet. Countless research has shown that fats help maintain and even increase testosterone levels. Omega-3s, monounsaturated, and even saturated fats in diet have all shown to increase testosterone levels.

Quality, consistent sleep. Your body can't recuperate its hormone levels if you don't get at least eight hours of uninterrupted sleep. People who work swing shifts or change the times of day they sleep constantly also throw their hormones out of balance.

Long-term dieting. When you are in a calorie deficit, you release cortisol and lower your testosterone levels. It also lowers other hormones such as the thyroid. During dieting, people generally aren't as healthy or energetic.

Don't overtrain. Excessive weight training and other exercise like cardio eventually lead to a gradual build-up of cortisol and lowering of testosterone.

Prescription/over-the-counter drugs. Find out if a prescription drug or over-the-counter drug interferes with testosterone or DHT. Some drugs for hair loss (Nizoral, Proscar, etc.) block or interfere with the conversion of testosterone to DHT and may cause side effects since DHT is more responsible for masculinizing sex effects than testosterone in males.

Zinc. A few years ago, zinc was shown to boost testosterone levels in football athletes when taken together with vitamin B6. This led to the ZMA craze among bodybuilders, which was a proprietary blend of zinc and vitamin B6. Zinc prevents the conversion of testosterone to DHT, helping to maintain healthy testosterone levels. It is also good for the prostate and, if taken before bed, very helpful for getting a good deep sleep.

Most people are deficient to some degree in zinc. You can supplement with extra zinc even beyond your multivitamin. Taking ZMA specifically is not necessary for the benefits of zinc as vitamin B6 only helps aid in zinc's absorption.

6-OXO. An anti-oestrogen supplement developed by the well-known bodybuilding supplement chemist Patrick Arnold. Anti-oestrogen supplements available on the market today help boost natural testosterone production by lowering the oestrogen in your body. They should be safe for those over twenty-one as long as it is for brief occasional cycles. Unlike steroids, they do not shut down testosterone production or create supraphysiological levels many times that of natural levels. Instead, they increase testosterone levels to a level moderately higher than you normally would have. When you get off anti-oestrogens, your testosterone levels will decrease again as your body goes back to equilibrium.

Warmer weather. I've come across studies that showed that in the cooler months, men's testosterone levels dropped. I'm sure there is a genetic basis for this, so living in warmer weather most of the year is an advantage for maintaining testosterone levels.

Lower body fat percentage. The higher your body fat percentage is, most likely the lower your testosterone levels will go. Your fat cells aromatize testosterone to oestrogen instead of DHT. Oestrogen in the body tends to decrease natural testosterone levels.

Exercise regularly. Exercise helps keep your testosterone and other hormones at healthy levels; just don't overtrain.

I hope you learned from this how to effectively increase your testosterone levels. This is the list I've compiled after reading research studies and bodybuilding articles for years.

17. The Health Benefits of Juicing

Juicing is one of the best ways to compensate for the toxins and ever-diminishing nutrient value of our food. For some people, whipping fresh fruits and vegetables through a juicer and extracting a glassful of vitamin-packed nectar ensure that they get the recommended five to seven servings of these foods every day. Others like juicing to get more carotenoids and flavonoids, which are healing compounds that can fight major diseases like cancer and heart disease. Still others see juicing as a way to get rid of the toxins in the body, boost immunity, and help to treat a variety of diseases, like anaemia, constipation, and arthritis.

Juices are a multivitamin/mineral supplement for people who don't want to take pills and capsules. Your body absorbs the nutrients much better than it does from pills. Although plants are full of vitamins, minerals, and other healing compounds, these substances are bound to fibrous tissue and contained within cellulose walls. When you grind up vegetables or fruits to make juice, you break down the cellulose, releasing these compounds and making them available for absorption.

Unless you chew very, very well, you won't get all the nutrients from food that you get from juice. In fact, juice is one of the most powerful whole foods that you can put in your body. It takes very little energy to digest it, so you maintain almost all the energy and nutrients that it gives. Plus, it takes a whole lot of vegetables to get the same amount of nutrients found in one glass of juice.

A 6-ounce glass of carrot juice contains large amounts of beta-carotene, which, when it's converted to vitamin A in the body, is 948 per cent of the daily value. The same glass of juice also contains 16 milligrams of vitamin C, 27 per cent of the daily value; 0.4 milligram of vitamin B6, or 20 per cent of the daily value; 537 milligrams of potassium, or 15 per cent of the DV; and 0.2 milligram of thiamine, or 11 per cent of the daily value.

Juicing can even help to control your weight. Drinking juices helps the body iron out its nutritional deficiencies, which leaves you more satisfied from a healthy diet and less likely to overeat.

Despite their nutritional goodness, juices should be used to supplement fresh fruits, vegetables, and grains in your diet, not to replace them. Juices don't contribute much toward the 20 to 35 grams of fibre that adults need each day.

For example, eight carrots provide 17 grams of fibre, while a 6-ounce glass of juice contains a measly 2 grams.

Fresh juices supply more than the necessary vitamins and minerals. They also contain a variety of phytonutrients. If you have read my article, 'Phytochemicals, Compounds to Cut Cancer and Heart Disease', you would know it already.

Perhaps the best known of the phytonutrients is beta-carotene, a plant pigment that gives the orange colour on sweet potatoes and carrots and the red on tomatoes.

Fruit and vegetables also contain flavonoids, compounds that have strong antioxidant power and prevent low-density-lipoprotein (LDL) cholesterol. You can read all about flavonoids in my article 'Flavonoids, Powerful Antioxidants to Prevent Cancer and Heart Disease' and also 'Healthy for Life with Digestive Enzymes'.

In a large study of more than 100,000 people, researchers found that adding one serving of fruits and vegetables to the diet each day lowered the risk of ischemic stroke, a stroke in which the artery to the brain is blocked by 6 per cent.

The best protection came from citrus fruits, dark-green leafy vegetables, and cruciferous vegetables, which include broccoli, cauliflower, and cabbage.

Other studies have shown that antioxidants help prevent Alzheimer's disease. In 2002, researchers studied nearly 5,500 people and found that those who ate diets rich in the antioxidant vitamins C and E lowered their risk of developing Alzheimer's disease. Drinking a large variety of vegetable and fruit juices is a wonderful way to get therapeutic amounts of all these healing compounds.

Drink your juices right away; otherwise, it will lose their nutritional benefits, and the flavour is also fleeting. Some juices, like cabbage, become funky in a few hours. So it's best to make only as much as you plan to drink right away.

Focus on vegetables. While a tall glass of fruit juice may appeal to you, it's better to concentrate on vegetable juices. Fruit juices are high in sugar and too acidic to drink in large quantities. Vegetable juices are better nutritionally. For maximum healing benefits, drink vegetable juices from a variety of vegetables. The more variety you can put into your diet, the better.

18. The Health Benefits of Tea

Tea stops tumours causing heart disease and stroke, according to laboratory studies. And as it contains clout, it protects against dental cavities.

Also, hundreds of compounds in tea, called polyphenols, act as antioxidants. Meaning, they help neutralize harmful oxygen molecules in the body known as free radicals, which have been linked to cancer, heart disease, and various less serious problems, such as wrinkles.

'In General polyphenols are very good antioxidants. But tea contains the best polyphenols, and tea has a lot of them,' according to Joe A. Vinson, PHD, professor of analytical chemistry at the University of Scranton in Pennsylvania. 'They make up nearly 30% of tea's dry weight.' This may help explain why tea is the most popular beverage in the world.

Protection of Arteries

The results of blocked arteries, high blood pressure, heart attacks, and stroke don't happen overnight. Years of steadily increasing damage are proceeding, in which dangerous low-density-lipoprotein (LDL) cholesterol oxidizes and gradually makes arteries stiff and narrow.

Tea can solve this problem. Polyphenols in tea are extremely effective in preventing cholesterol from oxidizing blood vessels. In fact, one of the polyphenols in tea, epigallocatechin (EGCG), was able to neutralize five times as much LDL cholesterol as vitamin C, the strongest of the antioxidant vitamins.

Why are the polyphenols in tea so effective? The reason is because they can work in two ways. They block the harmful effects of oxidized LDL cholesterol in the bloodstream and at the artery walls, where LDL really produces atherosclerosis, says Dr Vinson.

Researchers from a Dutch study, involving 880 men, found that those who ate the most flavonoids, a large phytochemical family, including polyphenol in tea, had a 58 per cent lower risk of dying from heart disease than those who ate the least. After further analysing the results, it was revealed that the healthiest men were those who were getting more than half their flavonoids from black tea, and the rest from onions and apples.

You don't have to drink lots of tea to get the benefits. In the Dutch study, the healthiest men drank about four cups of tea per day.

Just as the tea protect arteries leading from the heart, the same effect happens on arteries in or leading to the brain, says Dr Vinson.

A new Japanese study found that people who drank at least five cups of green tea daily had a whopping 62 per cent lower risk of having a stroke from clotting arteries.

According to experts, antioxidants in green tea help sticky cells that clump together to form clots, called platelets, to slide safely past one another.

When there are no clots, there can be no strokes.

Cancer Protection

When you grill a hamburger, compounds called heterocyclic amines are formed on the surface of the food. The body transforms these chemicals into more dangerous forms, which can cause cancer, according to John Weisburger, MD, PhD, vice president for research and director of the Naylor Dana Institute for Disease Prevention in New York.

Other compounds found in tea, called polyphenols, prevent the formation of potential carcinogens, Dr Weisburger says. In other words, they help stop cancer before it starts.

Skin Cancer Protection

Cancer researcher Hasan Mukhtar, PhD, of the department of dermatology at the University of Wisconsin in Madison, has seen tea stopping cancer at each stage of its life cycle, arresting both its growth and spread. And where cancerous tumours have already formed, he has seen tea shrink them.

Dr Mukhtar studied the effect of sunburn skin on laboratory animals and found that the animals given tea developed one-tenth as many tumours as those given water.

Even when the tea-given animals developed tumours, they were often benign, not cancerous. What's more, tea was equally effective whether given as a drink or applied to the skin.

Some cosmetics companies have started adding green tea to skin products for its potential protective benefits.

Dental Protection

Tea also helps prevent toothache since it contains many compounds, polyphenols, as well as tannin that act as antibiotics. In other words, tea removes the bacteria that promote tooth decay. Tea also contains fluoride, which provides further dental protection. When researchers at Forsyth Dental Centre in Boston tested a variety of foods for their antibacterial qualities, they found that tea was far and away the most protective.

Researchers at Kyushu University in Fukuoka, Japan, have identified four components in tea—tannin, catechin, caffeine, and tocopherol (a vitamin E-like substance)—that help to increase the acid resistance of tooth enamel. This quartet of compounds was made even more effective with the addition of extra fluoride. The extra boost made tooth enamel 98 per cent impervious to the action of acids on the teeth.

Different Colours of Tea

You can have green tea, black tea, vanilla maple tea, raspberry tea, black currant tea, and apricot tea. Which tea has the most healing polyphenols?

It makes no difference as long as it is real tea and not herbal tea, which doesn't contain leaves from the *Camellia sinensis*, the tea plant. There is not much difference among them. They all contain leaves from the same plant.

However, they are not identical. The lightest leaves, green and white, are minimally processed and, in general, retain more disease-protective polyphenols and other antioxidants. But darker teas contain healthy theaflavins, which form when their polyphenols ferment and turn orange red.

Here follows an overview of the various 'real' teas.

Black. The colour refers to the leaves; the beverage is deep amber. Black tea varieties include Darjeeling and Earl Grey; flavours range from spicy to flowery. Black tea may lower the risk of heart disease and colon cancer; it can also inhibit bacteria that cause cavities and bad breath.

Green. If you find the flavour too 'grassy', try jewel green matcha or Japanese sencha. Green tea has been shown in numerous studies to help prevent many kinds of cancer, lower cholesterol, and boost immunity.

Oolong. Midway between green and black tea in colour, flavour, and antioxidant action, oolong has a fresh floral or fruity aroma. When you drink three cups a day, it may help relieve itchy skin rashes.

Pu-ehr (poo-air). This dark-red tea has an earthy flavour reminiscent of coffee and tobacco. It's considered a delicacy in China (you can purchase it online), where it's processing is a highly guarded secret. The most oxidized of teas, pu-ehr is said to mellow and improve with age, like wine. It may help reduce cholesterol.

White. Rare and somewhat expensive, the least processed tea has an extremely subtle flavour. But it does contain more antioxidants than other teas.

Test-tube studies show that it can block DNA mutations (which trigger tumour formation). A study on rats discovered it prevented precancerous colon tumours.

How to Get the Most Steep for Three Minutes

It takes three minutes for it to release the health-promoting compounds. That's also the time researchers use in their studies on tea. Longer steeping causes the tea to go bitter.

Use Teabags

The pulverized content of teabags release more polyphenols than the larger loose leaves. That's because the tiny particles in the bag yield more surface area for polyphenols to dissolve into hot water.

Choose Your Flavours

Although green tea has been more thoroughly researched than the black variety, both kinds show equally salutary effects, says Dr Vinson. If you prefer decaffeinated tea, that's okay. The removal of caffeine has little effect on tea's polyphenol content.

The same holds for bottled teas, iced tea, and tea made from mixes. In fact, some soft drinks and juice companies have been so impressed with the benefits of tea that they have begun fortifying their beverages with green tea. Check out your health food store for new products.

Don't use milk—at least for now. According to an Italian study, adding milk to tea, as the British do, blocked tea antioxidant benefits. 'There is some evidence that milk protein binds to some of the tea compounds and blocks their absorption. But those compounds could get unbound in the stomach. So we're not so sure milk is bad,' says Dr Vinson.

Keep it Fresh

When making your own iced tea, drink it within a few days. 'And make sure you cover it to keep it fresh when you refrigerate it,' he advises.

When you keep iced tea for longer than a week, the concentration of compounds falls off. Many bottled and powdered iced teas remain spectacular antioxidant levels.

In one prevention magazine analyses of antioxidants in various commercial iced teas, even the lowest-scoring convenience iced teas contained at least as many antioxidants as fruits and vegetables, such as strawberries and spinach! But highest honour went to home-made iced tea—cold-brewed refrigerator and classic hot-brewed tea that was then chilled came in even with each other for antioxidant levels. (One tip: shake cold-brewed tea before removing teabags. It seems to knock more antioxidants into the liquid.)

Drink Tea after Eating Meat

Because polyphenol compounds in tea help to block the formation of cancer-causing chemicals, it's a good idea to have a cup of tea after eating fried or charred meat.

Doctor's Top Tip

When you are a sneezer, drink more green tea. It may be useful against a wide range of sneeze-starting allergens, including pollen, pet dander, and dust. Go for two to three mugs a day.

Chapter 3

19. The Importance of Detoxification

The detoxification of your body should be your primary goal.

Although it is sometimes not the most pleasant phase of creating an environment for weight loss, it is necessary. If detoxification is too fast, it can create discomfort.

The building up of toxic waste in your body may have taken twenty up to fifty years or more, so detoxification is not something that is achieved overnight. It is absolutely essential for your system to be cleaned so that energy comes free to be used to reduce weight. As long as there is toxic waste in your system, much of your energy will be used to eliminate it. The success of any weight loss program depends on your system being cleaned. Detoxification is cleansing, which is the key to it all.

The possible degree of discomfort depends on how toxic your system is. People with a high level of toxicity or have taken drugs, on a regular basis, are more likely to experience some temporary discomfort than those who are less toxic. The elimination of toxic wastes can be uncomfortable.

It's important for a person's diet to be such that cleansing can take place, but not at breakneck speed.

The most frequent possible discomfort is bloating of the system as the application of the principle of eating fruit on an empty stomach till 12 a.m. can stir up toxic wastes, creating gas and bloat. Generally, this bloating passes within forty-eight hours. The cleansing process of fruit washes impacted faecal matter from the intestinal walls and flushes it out of the system in the form of loose stools. You may also experience nausea as the toxins in your system are stirred up.

The total elimination of all toxicity from your body can take months or years, but within days, you will lose weight and feel enormously more energetic and vibrant. The ongoing elimination usually continues without any outward signs or discomforts.

The increase of fruits and vegetables in your diet can decrease the risk of cancer and heart disease. Antioxidants in fruits and vegetables not only neutralize free radicals but also increase your resistance to all kinds of toxins.

Sugar's quick absorption into your bloodstream causes an excess insulin burst from the pancreas. On reaching your liver, excess insulin, which is toxic, is converted to neutral triglycerides, which are the type of fats that are stored in all your adipose cells. Eat complex carbohydrates instead of sugar.

Alu is a toxic metal and causes multiple forms of brain damage and is strongly linked with Alzheimer's disease. Eliminate it from your life in water cooking, utensils, antacids, and personal care products, like antiperspirants and shampoos. There are other toxic metals; Alu is just one of them.

Give your body a change to function it its highest possible level, unimpeded by toxic waste and overweight. Your body wants to shine; it does not want to be overweight.

It wants to have the shape you know it can have. All you have to do is make it easy for the natural processes to work properly, and you can start to enjoy the body you can be proud of.

You can eat well and enjoy your food. Avoid of putting yourself through those self-depriving two- or four-week ordeals that bring you nothing but frustration and temporary results. You now have a realistic, lifelong approach that you can live with—naturally!

20. How to Detox Your Body Naturally

Natural Hygiene

Natural hygiene is the most remarkable approach to the care and upkeep of the human body. Natural hygiene will teach you how to eat. The loss of weight is only one of the benefits of Natural hygiene as a lifestyle. A significant increase in energy and overall well-being is also one of the benefits of natural hygiene.

Natural hygiene is practiced today by people around the world who enjoy long, healthy, disease-free lives. The basic foundation of natural hygiene is that the body is always striving for health and that it achieves this by continuously cleansing itself of deleterious waste material.

It is the science of understanding the effect that food has on the length and quality of the life of a human being. Its focus is on prevention and healthful living. It teaches people how to eliminate the cause of their health problems rather than constantly battling the effects of continually violating natural laws.

The underlying basis of natural hygiene is that the body is self-cleansing, self-healing, and self-maintaining. It is based on the idea that all the healing power of the universe is in the human body that nature is always correct and cannot be improved upon.

When we talk about detoxing your body, we have to take note of the three natural body cycles.

Natural Body Cycles

These cycles are based on rather obvious functions of the human body. On a daily basis we take in food (appropriation), we absorb and use some of that food (assimilation), and we get rid of what we don't use (elimination).

Although each of these three functions is always going on to some extent, each is more intense during certain hours of the day.

1) Noon to 8 p.m.   Appropriation (eating and digestion)
2) 8 p.m. to 4 a.m.   Assimilation (absorption and use)
3) 4 a.m. to noon   Elimination (of body wastes and food debris)

Our body cycles can become apparent to us if we simply witness our bodies in action. Obviously, during the hours we are awake, we eat (appropriate), and if we put off eating, our hunger tends to increase as the day progresses.

When we are sleeping and the body has no other noticeable work to do, it is assimilating what was taken in during the day. When we awaken in the morning, we have what is called morning breath because our bodies are in the midst of eliminating of that which was not used—body wastes.

Physiologically, our bodies want to eat early in the evening so that at least three hours can pass, which is the time needed for food to leave the stomach and the assimilation cycle can start on time.

The reason that 62 per cent of the people in America are overweight is that our traditional eating habits have consistently violated the all-important elimination cycle.

In other words, we have been taking food in (at a record pace!), and we have been using what we need from that food, but we have *not* been getting rid of what we can't use. Far more time is spent appropriating than eliminating. So the secret of losing weight is to get rid of the toxic wastes and excesses we carry around.

Metabolic Imbalance

Natural hygiene uses the word *toxaemia* what modern science now calls metabolic imbalance. The human body is finely designed to stay in balance in terms of tissue building up (anabolism) and tissue breaking down (catabolism). An excess of one over the other is called metabolic imbalance.

By keeping your system toxin-free, you significantly increase your chance of having a comfortable body weight because excesses of toxins in the body are the forerunners of obesity.

Your body is building toxaemia daily in two ways: through the normal process of metabolism and by residue left over from the foods, which are not efficiently utilized.

As far as your weight is concerned, common sense will tell you that if more of this toxic waste is built than is eliminated, there is going to be a build-up of the excess. That translates to being overweight.

To make things worse, toxins are of an acid nature. When there is an acid build-up in the body, the system retains water to neutralize it, adding even more weight and bloat.

So how do we maintain metabolic balance and accomplish the removal of toxic waste from the system while still enjoying our food?

There are three easy-to-follow principles or tools that can assist you in doing just that. The first of these tools to help you realize your goal of *permanent* weight loss is the principle of high-water-content food.

The Principle of High-Water-Content Food

Water is important for our survival, and so is food and air. What do we mean when we talk about high-water-content food? Our earth we are living on contains 70 per cent water for survival. And so does our bodies. Maybe you find this hard to believe, but it's a fact. When you consider those two facts, wouldn't it make sense that to maintain a body that is always in top condition, you must consume a diet that also contains 70 per cent water?

If your body is 70 per cent water, so where does it get that water from if you don't replenish it on a regular basis? From the moment you are born until the last breath you take, your body is craving this essential of life.

This is besides drinking water. That's another subject. Drinking water does not bring the results I'm talking about.

When we talk about high-water-content food, there are only two types of food that have that high water content: they are fruits and vegetables. They should predominate in our diet.

Besides carrying nutrients into the body, water performs the essential function of cleansing the body of toxic wastes. All three of our body cycles function with the greatest ease when supplied with the water in fruits and vegetables on a regular basis.

If you want to be vibrantly and vigorously alive, in the best possible shape, you have to eat food that's alive.

The importance of proper food combining has been proved as a result of intense research over the last 100 years.

Food combining teaches us that the human body is not designed to digest more than one concentrated food in the stomach at the same time. Any food that is not a fruit or a vegetable is concentrated.

The principle of correct food combining is based on eleven different food groups and associated individual foods. You can get a food combining chart from 'Laugh with Health' from the Internet.

Another important thing to keep in mind is that drinking any liquid during a meal will upset the natural digestive process of the juices in the stomach. You should not drink within an hour before a meal or within two hours after a meal.

Most people like fruit but don't know how and when to eat it. The correct consumption of fruit is closely associated with proper food combining. Fruit is, without doubt, the most beneficial energy-giving food you can eat.

Fruit has the highest water content of any food. Fruit requires less energy to be digested than any other food, in fact, almost none. Fruit is glucose in the body. Fruit does not digest in the stomach. It is essential to eat it on an empty stomach, and you should never eat it with or immediately following anything else. This is also very important. Fruit is the most important food that you can eat.

How long do you have to wait before you can eat fruit? This depends on the type of food. After a salad or raw vegetables, you have to wait two hours.

After a properly combined meal without meat—3 hours

After a properly combined meal with meat—4 hours

After any improperly combined meal—8 hours

From the time you wake up in the morning till noon, eat *only* fresh fruit and fruit juice. When you eat fresh fruit on an empty stomach, it has only a positive effect; it accelerates weight loss.

21. Diet and Weight Loss

If you are looking for some practical advice for weight loss and keep it off permanently, the following information will help you to achieve this.

For weight loss, five days weekly exercise of thirty minutes is much superior to three days weekly of seventy minutes, even though the total weekly exercise time of the three-day people is an hour longer. In order to keep that metabolic rate churning, frequent exercise is the key.

For healthy, permanent weight loss, depriving yourself is not the answer. Deprivation and bingeing become a vicious circle, and that's just one of the many problems with dieting.

Another thing is that diets are temporary; therefore, the results have to be temporary. The fact of the matter is that dieting doesn't work. It never has, and it never will.

If diets worked, would the rate of obesity in America not decrease each year instead of increase? In 1982, fifteen billion dollars was spent on weight-loss schemes in the US alone!

If diets worked, that incredible high amount of money would surely put an end to this problem, wouldn't it? The fact is that this ridiculous high amount is increasing by one billion dollars every year. In spite of the new diets that come and go, the problem is becoming worse.

Facts about Fat Storage

The industry around weight loss is well aware of the fact that low-calorie diets cause fast loss of muscle and fat. For this reason, the market is saturated with fibre bars, liquid meals, and lightweight cereals.

We live in a society of instant coffee, while-you-wait, etc. Fast results are essential for continuous sales results. The average consumer is not aware of the fact that when they are losing fat, they lose muscle also.

Nutrition scientists have known for many years that reducing calories to 800–1,200 per day, which is below the essential energy requirement of the body to maintain vital functions, causes you to cannibalize your own muscles for fuel.

On these diets, muscle provides up to 45 per cent of the energy deficit. If the deficit in essential energy requirement is 500 calories per day, then up to 225 calories will come from muscle breakdown. In only four weeks on such a diet, you can lose 1.5 kilograms of vital muscle. In your muscles is all your energy created by burning of fats, carbohydrates, and proteins in the mitochondria of every cell.

Even an ounce of muscle lost lowers basic metabolic rate of fuel consumption and reduces your ability to burn body fat. So, all diets that are below the essential energy requirement of your body are a guaranteed recipe for failure.

Besides the fact of losing muscle, which is your body's engine, the weight loss industry also knows that fast fat loss guarantees regain of fat. The physiology behind it has been known for decades.

Fast fat loss alerts the potent defences of the body of its energy reserve.

The quantity and activity of the lipoprotein lipase enzyme increase immediately, which is the body's main mechanism that collect digested fat from the bloodstream and stuff it into fat cells.

Lipoprotein lipase get hold of every fat molecule and even disable your body to use it for energy. In order to make up the deficit, you have to burn more muscle.

However, as muscle is your basic structure, it is harder for your body to burn it than fat. As a result, your metabolism slows down, which reduces your ability to burn fat. Toxic wastes build up as a result of burning proteins. This can make you sick and cranky.

This activity does not help you to control your appetite, which becomes more ravenous. It gets even worse. If you can't resist the inconvenience any longer and succumb to real food, the lipoprotein lipase has become so efficient that you regain seven weeks' painful fat loss in almost seven days.

But the biggest problem is that you don't get any of the lost muscle back. So, the final result of the diet is that there is no change in body fat but a big loss in muscle. This loss of part of your engine causes further fat gain as it reduces your ability to burn the fat you have.

Overweight people using low-calorie diets lose so much muscle that they set their bodies up for permanent obesity, when they use them repeatedly.

22. Following a Low-Fat Diet for Good Health

The subject of my last article was low-carb diets. Another way to reduce weight is to follow a low-fat diet. It has been proven during the last few decades that reducing the amount of saturated fat in your body is one of the best things you can do for your health.

Fatty foods will significantly increase your risk of heart disease, diabetes, high blood pressure, certain types of cancer, and many other conditions. Today, 66 per cent of Americans are overweight or obese, and the rate of obesity has more than doubled to 32 per cent, with most of the increase happening during the past twenty years.

Reducing the total calorie intake is the key to losing weight. And to eat less fat is the easiest way to do that. One gram of fat delivers nine calories, which is more than twice as many as the same amount of protein or carbohydrate. Also, our body likes fat. It's easier to store calories from fat than from other sources.

In one study, Danish researchers found that those who reduced the amount of fat in their diets from 39 per cent to 28 per cent of total calories and increased their intake of carbohydrates were able to lose an average of nine pounds in just twelve weeks. In addition, people who stuck to lower-fat diets were able to keep the weight off long after the study ended.

According to research, another advantage of reducing fat from your diet is that it can increase your general sense of well-being. In a study of more than 550 women, researchers at the Fred Hutchinson Cancer Research Centre in Seattle found that when the women cut their daily fat intake in half from 40 per cent to 20 per cent of total calories, they felt more vigorous, less anxious, and less depressed than they had when they were eating their former diets.

Heart health fat in your diet often goes to your arteries. There is a direct link between the amount of fat in your diet and your risk for heart disease. This is particularly true of saturated fat, the dangerous type that can clog your arteries and we find mainly in meats, full-fat dairy products, and snack foods. Research has shown that eating a diet low in saturated fat is the best way to lower this risk.

You don't have to go on an extremely low-fat diet to get the benefits. Even reducing the amount of saturated fat in your diet just a little bit can lead to a reduction in cholesterol levels.

Cancer Protection

Making the switch to a low-fat diet offers great protection against many diseases, including cancer. Researchers at the University of Benin in Nigeria found that when laboratory animals were fed high-fat diets, they began producing enzymes that led to cancerous changes in their colons in just three weeks.

What works in the laboratory can also be applied in real life. In a study of 450 women, researchers in the department of epidemiology and public health at Yale University School of Medicine found that cutting just 10 grams of saturated fat a day—the equivalent of switching from two glasses of whole milk to the same amount of fat-free milk—could reduce the risk of ovarian cancer by 20 per cent.

A low-fat diet is protective not only because of what it doesn't contain but also because of what it does. When you cut back on fats, you generally eat more fruits, vegetables, whole grains, and legumes, all of which have been shown to keep us healthier, says JoAnn Manson, MD, professor of women's health at Brigham and Women's Hospital in Boston.

Good for the eyes to close it off. Eating a low-fat diet may also protect you against macular degeneration, which is the leading cause of vision loss in older adults. In a survey of more than 2,000 people, researchers from the University of Wisconsin in Madison found that those who reported getting the most saturated fat had 80 per cent higher risk of getting macular degeneration than those getting the least.

Start your low-fat diet. If you want to start reducing the amount of fat in your diet, it's not always easy to know where to begin. Firstly, you have to find out how much fat you're actually getting each day. Ideally, you should get between 25 per cent and 30 per cent of your total calories from fat.

For example, suppose you normally get 2,000 calories per day. When you're following a low-fat diet, no more than 600 of your total calories should come from fat. This will add up to 67 grams of fat per day.

Don't let lowering your fat intake to 30 per cent discourage you! This is a reasonable amount of fat to go into your diet. According to Lalita Kaul, PhD, a national spokesperson for the American Dietetic Association and professor of nutrition at the Medical School of Howard University in Washington, DC, eating low fat means avoiding fried foods; forgoing rich, fatty restaurant meals for home-cooked fare; and searching for tasty low-fat recipes with which to replace some of your higher-fat favourites. Reach for a Lean Cuisine meal or a Lean Pocket when you're looking for at-home convenience.

Probably the easiest way to keep track of your daily fat intake is reading food labels. They are based on a 2,000-calorie diet. So, you can look at foods which are 30 per cent or below. To avoid partially hydrogenated oils, look for a spread that says 'zero trans fat' on the label. And avoid cookies and other baked goods and snack foods that contain trans fats. Trans fats are now required to be listed on nutrition labels along with total and saturated fat. If you are dining out or buy foods that don't have labels, you can buy a nutrition reference guide in a bookstore or supermarket.

As mentioned before, the most dangerous type of fat to watch out for is saturated fat, which is found in animal foods like meat, butter, cheese, and eggs, and some plant sources such as coconut oil, palm oil, tropical oils, and cocoa butter. The same foods that are high in saturated fat are also high in cholesterol. So, when you decrease one, you automatically decrease the other.

The American Heart Association recommends that we should get less than 7 per cent of our total calories from saturated fat, partly by choosing fat-free or low-fat milk and leaner cuts of meat, like sirloin or top round.

Enjoy the good fats in moderation generally. You should reduce all kind of fats in your diet. Although monounsaturated and polyunsaturated fats are not bad, you should eat them in moderation because they contain as many calories as bad fats. They are found in vegetable and seed oils, such as olive, sesame, and safflower oils, and in nuts and seeds. They have been shown to actually lower cholesterol and may help prevent it from sticking to artery walls.

The fat found in fish, omega-3 fatty acids, has been shown to reduce clotting and inflammation in the arteries, which can significantly reduce the risk of heart disease and stroke. You don't have to eat a lot of fish to get the benefits. When you're following a low-fat diet, having two fish meals a week will go a long way toward keeping your arteries in the swim.

23. Antioxidant Protection

Oxidation in our body is the main cause of many forms of cancer, heart disease, atherosclerosis, adult-onset diabetes, cataracts, lung and liver disorders, and degenerative diseases of the brain and can be prevented and even reversed by the proper use of the right antioxidants.

According to the *Journal of the American Medical Association*, cancer is still on the rise. Dr Deva Davis and her colleagues confirmed that cancer increase is presumably the result from exposure to carcinogens in our environment, including pesticides, herbicides, chemical solvents, smoking, and industrial and auto emissions.

Smoking is the worst out of those mentioned. The damage is done mainly by oxidation and in combination with other air pollutants; it is the cause of 33 per cent of all cancers. Overweight follows as the next big cancer risk with 24 per cent.

The American Cancer Society began a massive study in 1959 involving more than one million people in twenty-five American states, which ended in 1980. The results showed that people who are 40 per cent or more overweight have higher rates of a wide variety of cancers.

Many of these cancers are caused by lipid oxidation. That means excess fat molecules in your body go rancid and initiate cell damage that develops into cancer.

For the average person, pesticides seem a bigger cancer threat than being overweight. Cancer risk from too much body fat is much higher than all the pesticides together.

24. Nutritional Supplements

It's not easy to eat the recommended 1 to 2 cups of fruits, 2 to 3 cups of vegetables, and 3 to 4 ounces of grains every day.

We are living in a fast-paced age, spending too many lunch times rushing through fast-food lines. Then we drive to the supermarket or pharmacy, where we stock-up on vitamins, minerals and food extracts in the hope that these pills will help us to get the all-important nutrients when our diets fail to supply them.

But is there really any value in taking these supplements? According to Mary Ellen Camire, PhD, professor in the department of food science and human nutrition at the University of Maine in Orono, they certainly can! 'When you're running around and skipping meals, taking a multivitamin can help you get nutrients that you may be missing.'

It's a fact that many doctors now believe that supplements may do more than make up for deficiency in nutrition. There is evidence that even if you're eating well, supplements can make you healthier. Michael Jansen, MD, author of Dr Janson's New Vitamin Revolution says: 'The scientific literature clearly states that people who get certain nutrients, like vitamins C and E, in higher levels than you can get from foods are going to get additional benefits.'

The federal Food and Nutrition Board, a committee of the National Academy of Science - National Research Council, which is made up of a prestigious group of nutritional scientists, has been telling us for more than 80 years, how much of various nutrients we should try to get from our food each day. The board's recommendations, called Recommended Dietary Allowances, prepared to act as guidelines for good basic nutrition. (A shorthand version of these recommendations, called Daily Values, or DV's, are the numbers that you can see on food labels.)

Lately, scientists started to find connections between vitamins and the prevention of some health threats that they didn't know before, including links to cancer and heart disease. Although the DV's are high enough to prevent deficiency diseases, such as rickets, scurvy and beri-beri, which used to be common problems in society, they may not be high enough to prevent other diseases that are more common today.

There is also a deficiency particularly in antioxidant vitamins C and E. These are essential to block the damaging effect of free radicals on healthy cells. They are thought to be the main cause of serious health conditions, like heart disease, cancer, dementia and others. Because free radicals are created in enormous quantities every day, the amounts of antioxidants recommended by the DV's may not be enough to neutralize the free radicals.

Another important nutrient that is lacking in the American diet is omega-3 fatty acids. Omega-3 are "essential" fatty acids, meaning that our bodies can't make them. we must get them from our diet. Fish oil provides the most powerful omega-3.

Research has proved that omega-3 found in fatty fish, canola oil, flaxseed, and walnuts, among other foods, help prevent heart disease and cancer, improve joint health, and may even be protective against depression and dementia. Unfortunately, Americans get only about 25 per cent of the omega-3 we need every day. We should get a ratio of 4:1: 4 units of omega-6 against 1 unit omega-3. Omega-6 is another essential fatty acid found in grain.

The international agreed-upon recommendation of omega-3 is 650 milligram per day, which is hard to get from fish alone. Fortunately, there are quality fish oil supplements on the market. One of them is Nordie Naturals Omega-3 capsules. Take one capsule per day to boost your omega-3s.

Apart from omega-3 fatty acids, vitamin E is also an important nutrient, which comes in high fat foods like vegetable oils, nuts for example. When people reduce the amount of fat in their diet, they may also reduce the amount of vitamin E as well. A vitamin E supplement may help to reach your goal, without all the fat.

What are the amounts we need? The major antioxidants and their co-factors in the forms and amounts used by the Colgan Institute and other laboratories in studies that have successfully inhibited a wide variety of diseases, and have also improved the vitality and performance of people already in excellent health are as follows:

Some studies have proven that by eating a lot of fruits and vegetables high in vitamin C can help protect against numerous forms of cancer, including cancer of the pancreas, esophages, larynx, mouth, stomach, colon and rectum, cervix, breast and lungs. However, there is no evidence that support taking vitamin C supplements for cancer protection. Scientists believe the other phytochemicals in vitamin C-rich fruits and vegetables could play a role in the protection. When it comes to cancer protection, you may be better off sticking to foods to get your vitamin C.

Other studies have shown that taking amounts of vitamin C above and beyond the DV can boost immunity, improve lung function, and lower the risk of heart disease and cataracts. One Finnish study published in Stroke: The Journal of the American Heart Association showed that men with the lowest blood levels of vitamin C had more than two times the stroke risk of men with the highest blood levels of vitamin C. It seems that vitamin C may help prevent clogged arteries and lower blood pressure, making blood vessels more flexible.

Vitamin E is a very powerful antioxidant. Studies indicated that it may block the process that causes cholesterol to stick to artery walls, while at the same time preventing platelets, the blood components that can cause blood clotting, from clumping together in the bloodstream and increasing the risk of heart disease.

While supplements can work for some nutrients, the benefits are not so clear for beta-carotene. Although foods rich in beta-carotene, like carrots, spinach, and kale, have proved to help prevent a variety of illnesses, cancer included, beta-carotene supplements haven't shown to be as useful and may even be harmful. It appears that this nutrient may work best when it's taken combined with other protective plant compounds- in other words, when you get it in its natural form from foods. One sweet potato contains almost 15 milligrams of beta-carotene. Other good sources include bright orange and dark green vegetables, such as winter squash, collard greens, and broccoli. Also, fruits, such as cantaloupe and dried apricots.

Neutraceuticals When you are going to shop for vitamins and minerals, look for the neutraceuticals section of the store. Vitamin and mineral supplements contain some nutrients, but the so-called neutraceutical supplements contain compounds extracted from whole foods, which are then supposedly concentrated into a Jetson-like pill. You can find pills containing broccoli, spinach, tomatoes, mixed vegetables, fruit juices and more. The advantage of neutraceuticals is that they supposedly contain all of the compounds naturally found in foods in the same proportion that nature intended. It may sound too good to be true and most researchers think it is unrealistic to think that you can reduce foods down to pills and still can get all the benefits, and most studies confirm this. However, even if the pills provide all the health-protecting compounds and phytochemicals that you can get from fruits and vegetables, they probably won't contain the fibre, says Dr Camire. Also, the process of making the pills may damage some of the healthful chemicals they claim to contain. 'Mother Nature's chemicals are much more potent than the ones made in factories," she adds.

At the very least, however, fruits and vegetables in pill form may provide a bit of a boost for folks who are not always able to eat as well as they would like, or for people who dislike fruits and vegetables so much that they find it impossible to choke hem down. 'There are a lot of people out there who simply do not or will not eat vegetables.' Says Dr Camire. 'For these people, the pills may be somewhat beneficial.' Dr Camire note that it is important to read labels carefully. However, some products that call themselves neutraceuticals only contain one or two isolated extracts – of carotenoids, for example- and not the full complement of health-promoting compounds found in the real foods.

25. How to Protect Your Body against Cancer

1. Choose a balanced diet consisting of a variety of fresh fruits and vegetables (green, yellow, and red), approximately three-quarters of total food intake by weight, preferably organically grown, if possible. Include cruciferous vegetables (cabbage), carrots, tomatoes, and garlic.

2. Avoid the consumption of deep-fried food, overcooked food, saturated fat, and trans- fat.

3. Don't overeat. 'Let food be your medicine and medicine be your food.'

4. Choose unprocessed food, low in fat, preferably from plants, and avoid animal fats and hydrogenated oils, including margarine. Use fresh flaxseed oil or fish oil for omega-3 fatty acids.

5. Eat adequate protein from plant sources and fibre from vegetables, fruits, whole grains, nuts, legumes, seeds, oat bran, and rice bran.

6. Avoid toxic synthetic chemicals as much as possible, particularly pesticides and other toxic chemicals. Drink filtered water, preferably reverse osmosis, to avoid chlorine and heavy metals.

7. Increase intake of natural minerals and vitamins from the juices of green, yellow, and red vegetables. Supplement your diet with high-quality multiminerals and antioxidants, particularly carotenoids, zinc, selenium, and folic acid (vitamin B9).

8. Consume low-glycaemic food with a low glycaemic load and keep calorie intake low overall.

9. Minimize intake of caffeine, alcohol, white sugar, white flour, table salt (use sea salt instead), cured meats, and smoked foods.

10. Keep clear of radiation. Research shows that nearly three-quarters of the energy from the antenna of a mobile phone is absorbed by the head. This radiation is the same kind of energy from microwave ovens and is sought to create hotspots in the brain.

It's a well-known fact that x-rays are causing cancer, even diagnostic use. An Australian radiologist estimated that about 270 Australians die each year from cancer caused by such tests. Also, the electromagnetic radiation from power lines and household appliances may contribute slightly carcinogenic effects.

11. Exercise regularly, at least three times per week for half an hour. For example, brisk walking can make the necessary difference to an otherwise sedentary lifestyle.
12. Find ways to cope with stress, for example, by practicing meditation and yoga.

26. The Truth about Skin Cancer

Australia leads the world as the country with the highest rate of skin cancer; about 140,000 new cases of non-melanomic skin cancer occur every year. Melanoma, which is the most dangerous form, causes 800 deaths each year. The rate has doubled over the last 40 years, and the incidence of skin cancer has almost doubled in the last 10 years.

The victims are getting younger each year. According to the *Australian Journal of Public Health*, from 40 per cent to 70 per cent of teenagers have permanent skin damage to some degree.

We can recognize three types of skin cancer. (Sunspots, the most common of all skin diseases in Australia, are not cancer but may be proceeding real cancer.)

Basal Cell Carcinoma (BCC)
This is the least dangerous form. It rarely spreads to other parts of the body and is seldom fatal.

Squamous Cell Carcinoma (SCC)
This type is also common and seldom fatal. However, it has to be treated as soon as possible because it has a greater risk of spreading.

Malignant Melanoma (MM)

This is the rarest kind of skin cancer but the most dangerous. It behaves like an internal cancer and will spread to other parts of the body and has to be treated early.

In the beginning stage, it looks like a mole, unusual freckle, or a birthmark. Warning signs are changes in colour, texture, size, or shape. It can bleed or become sore.

The current skin cancer rates have reached epidemic proportions and are caused by ultraviolet radiation, which is more intense in areas where there is a hole in the ozone layer. As the hole gets larger and presumably the rest of the layer gets thinner, more UV rays reach the earth's surface, including the very dangerous UVC radiation. As a result, our skin has to cope with an extra severe battering when we are outdoors.

We would expect skin cancer rates to be higher in Queensland, but the mortality rates from melanoma are higher in Tasmania and Brisbane. However, as the hole in the ozone layer sometimes reaches the Australian mainland and ozone thinning as far north as Brisbane, it is impossible to determine what the greater factor is: the ozone layer or the tropical sun.

Surprisingly, there is a higher number of people with melanoma among those who work indoors all year long compared to those who work outdoors all year.

This removes any doubt that other factors play a part in it as the incidence of melanoma is increasing on parts of the body least exposed to sunlight.

We can conclude that just over half of the present cases of melanoma can be explained as caused by the sun. Conventional wisdom can't explain the remainder.

There is strong evidence that melanoma (skin cancer in general) is yet another 'degenerative disease'. According to Professor Laura and John Aston in *Hidden Hazards* (Bantam Books 1991), sunlight is therapeutic and may help to prevent many diseases, including melanoma. Regular daily exposure to sunlight is an essential preventive measure, with the emphasis on *regular*.

This explains why indoor workers, who go out in the sun only occasionally, will not have developed the protective mechanisms, including pigmentation. But there are still other factors than just the sun.

These are environmental factors. The research of Ronald Laura and John Aston in their report from forty years ago, *Hidden Hazards*, revealed 100 substances had already been recognized as being photosensitizing agents.

These agents include many commonly used drugs, like some broad-spectrum antibiotics, tranquillizers, high blood pressure drugs, and drugs for hypoglycaemia. These also include some artificial sweeteners, including cyclamates. Deficiency of vitamin B6 refining removes much of the B6 from grains, with white bread containing one-fifth as much as wholemeal. Regarding synthetic riboflavin (vitamin B2), which is used extensively to fortify cereals, it appears that natural riboflavin does not sensitize the skin. Also included are ethyl alcohol, which is used in beverages; some synthetic chemicals, including solubilizers; and some fungicides and insecticides.

The paradox of skin cancer now seems to be resolved. Regardless the hole in the ozone layer, the appearance of artificial chemicals in recent years that sensitize the skin to light exactly explains the explosion in skin cancer incidence.

We don't need to be in the tropics to be at risk. By using these chemicals, we increase our accessibility wherever we are.

There are also hormonal factors. 'The effect of light on the regulation of our hormonal system appears to have the greatest potential for explaining the melanoma enigma,' say Professor Laura and John Ashton.

The existence of oestrogen receptors in melanoma cells may explain why oral contraceptives may increase the risk of melanoma, underscoring the important role of female sex hormones.

Also, the ovulatory cycle is regulated by light, both light entering the eyes, which influences the pineal gland, and light falling on the skin.

Artificial light, which is inadequate and incomplete compared to natural light, tends to hinder these light-dependent mechanisms, which lead ultimately to the production in the skin of the protective pigment: melanin.

Another unexpected effect of deprivation of natural light has been found in UV radiation to increase the cholesterol content of the skin. Both light entering the eyes and light falling on the skin regulate blood cholesterol levels. The higher cholesterol content provides greater protection against the effects of the radiation, with less risk of tumour formation.

Research has also raised the possibility that unnatural fat, like polyunsaturated margarines, affects the fat composition of the skin, disturbing the balance of the above-mentioned mechanisms, thereby explaining another factor that can cause melanoma.

There is strong evidence that vitamin D stimulates the entire hormone system to protect against melanoma and other cancers. It is important to know that vitamin D is made in the body, both when sunlight falls on the skin and when it enters the eyes, to regulate pineal function.

An Australian study revealed that working under fluorescent light doubles the risk of melanoma. Contrary to this, when sunlight strikes the skin, the UVB component in particular stimulates melanin production, which gives remarkable resistance against the damaging effect of ultraviolet radiation.

It has been proposed that very moderate exposure to sunlight every day during late winter and spring might provide enough protective melanin to withstand the intense UV radiation during summer.

Chapter 4

27. Fitness

Fitness can look long, complicated, tedious and, for some seemingly impossible to achieve. Fitness—and the lack of it—is the result of multiple small daily choices made over time. Every choice is a chance to move one step closer to thriving. Fitness is the ideal, so many people put a focus on health, which is more of a form of general wellness and may seem easier to achieve. But health is a funny thing—when we are young and healthy, we neither notice it nor think much about it.

However, health brings a freedom that few people realize until they no longer have it. I read a quote somewhere that goes something like this: "A healthy person has 1,000 dreams. The unhealthy person has one." There is much wisdom in this. If you are healthy, you have a myriad of things you are doing and planning to do. When you talk to an unhealthy person, you most often hear only about what's wrong with their health.

A lack of vitality has a narrowing effect on your perspective. It makes life seem less hopeful and less full of opportunity to experience the things we value.

Slowing Down the Aging Clock

Imagine you are a caveman or cave woman in a tribe of 20 people. Resources are scarce at times and survival is the highest priority. As such, it is important that more resources go to children and adults of reproductive age. Over time, this scenario has been built into our DNA on a deep level. There are triggers in our bodies that start the process of winding down toward the end of life. You can, however, fool that system a little bit.

If you remain physically active, you are still contributing to the resources of the tribe (through building shelter, hunting, gathering, etc.) Your body doesn't know you live in modern times. If you're moving a lot and in challenging enough ways, you're still doing your part to contribute, so your body maintains itself more effectively and for longer.

How We Weaken with Age

Weakness with aging comes from deterioration of myelin around muscle and a lower number of motor nerves, but vigorous exercise counteracts this process. The myelin is like insulation around electrical wires, and your motor nerves are those electrical wires. The signals sent on those wires are how your brain makes your muscles move and apply the right amount of force to do whatever you are asking it to do.

For the brain itself, reactive, coordinated physical activity does far more to promote brain health than "traditional" exercise, which is controlled, discrete movements like pedaling on a stationary bike. All exercise enhances brain health, but the right type of exercise protects the brain from future damage and enhances its function now. Running outdoors, catching a ball, interactive, partner-based workouts, playing a sport—even at a leisurely pace—are all more reactive and unpredictable, which enhances the brain benefits of physical activity.

Eye of the Tiger…or Alley Cat

Here's the best part: You can shift to thriving rather than just surviving today—right now. Your body and brain change based on what you do, big and small, moment to moment, and that adds up to significant change over time.

Direct the "eye of the tiger" toward your health choices and you'll thrive. Use the "eye of the alley cat" and you'll just get by and survive. Keep your "eye of the tiger" alive by making small choices each day related to your nutrition and physical activity that nudge you closer to health and fitness. You just might end up with a group of schoolkids chanting "Flex! Flex! Flex!" to you when you're 67 years old.

Get better or just get by. Survive or thrive. The next opportunity to choose is coming soon.

The human body is designed for activity, to obtain fitness. The coach potato lifestyle of the vast majority of our society during the last century has been an unnatural phenomenon. Physical activity was a regular feature of our ancestors. However, due to the change in lifestyle from agriculturalists to an industrialized and sedentary lifestyle, there has been a corresponding shift in our physical make up.

The benefits of physical activity in order to improve our body's functioning and composition can't be underestimated. Regular physical exercise to improve your fitness results in the following beneficial effects:

1. It elevates your metabolism.
2. It increases your aerobic capacity.
3. It maintains, tones, and strengthens your muscles.
4. It lowers your risk of heart disease.

5. It reduces diabetes risk.
6. It improves mental health.
7. It slows down some effects of aging.
8. It increases your HDL level.
9. It reduces the risk of death from leading causes.
10. It increases heart efficiency and lowers the heart rate.
11. It reduces the risk of developing osteoporosis.
12. It reduces the risk of developing many forms of cancer.
13. It reduces the pain associated with pregnancy.
14. It reduces ulcer risk.
15. It increases the number of red blood cells and their oxygen-carrying capacity.
16. It increases the production of new blood vessels in the heart and other muscles.
17. It improves sleep patterns.
18. It increases cartilage thickness.
19. It increases blood flow to the skin.
20. It increases alertness.
21. It improves pasture.
22. It improves immune system functioning.
23. It gives relief from mental stress.
24. It reduces lower back pain and the risk of lower back injury.
25. It maintains good overall function of the body.

Activity is a medicine for creating change in a person's physical, emotional, and mental states! All rewards are from doing, not knowing!

28. Activity: Protection Against All Diseases

Activity is important to **maintain a healthy body and for protection against all diseases.**

When you are not sleeping your body was designed to be almost continually active. If you immobilize a limb for just three hours, **it starts to degenerate.** That's why even during sleep you automatically flex and stretch and turn more than a hundred times in one night. Inactivity is deadly!

You can read this in a report by **Dr Walter Bortz** in the Journal of the American Medical Association in 1982. He reviewed over a hundred studies showing that the sedentary lifestyle developed in the last 50 years in America causes widespread bodily damage. This damage occurs independently of other health risk factors, like smoking, alcohol, fat, age and family history of disease.

Here follows some of his findings:

By itself, simple inactivity causes a chain reaction of **cardiovascular decay.** First, it reduces vital capacity. That means, sitting like a slug reduces your ability to take up and use oxygen. As a result, muscles, organs, and brain become partially oxygen deprived. In addition, inactivity reduces cardiac output, that is, the ability of your heart to pump blood around the body.

So the tissues of couch potatoes become double deprived. They get less oxygen and less blood and the essential nutrients the blood contains. In an effort to make up these deficits, your body constricts arteries, thereby **raising blood pressure.** This arterial constriction on top of a weakened heart not only increases the **risk of clots and stroke,** but also makes your **cardiovascular system less able to respond** to sudden movement or changes of position.

Consequently, sedentary folk often suffer dizziness on standing, because the impaired system cannot instantly increase blood flow to the brain. With any sudden movements they are prone to falls and accidents, because the restricted system of blood flow cannot respond efficiently.

One of the most interesting studies shows that more sedentary people than active people are hit and killed in traffic accidents. Because their weakened cardiovascular systems make them incapable of performing the nimble moves required to avoid oncoming traffic, without becoming dizzy and staggering or falling in the process.

Inactivity also increases levels of cholesterol and triglycerides. Triglycerides are the fats you store, and we know that inactivity makes you fat. Inactive muscles shrink, compromising your ability to burn fat, to perform even simple tasks, like running upstairs, and even to hold up your skeleton.

Bones also thin and weaken, because your skeleton requires continuous resistance exercise to be able to grow new bone matrix.

A combination of inactivity and poor bone nutrition is the major cause of the epidemic of osteoporosis now burdening America – another man made – entirely preventable disease.

Inactivity also disrupts bowel function and disorders glucose metabolism, independently of whatever food you eat. The near epidemics of intestinal disorders and adult-onset diabetes in America bear mute testimony to our slug lifestyle.

Sex hormone levels also decline with inactivity, now linked to the huge increase in impotence in America. The evidence is overwhelming that the incidence of male impotence in America has doubled since the 1940's.

Activity Can Save Your Life

One of the best studies was conducted by renowned exercise guru Dr. Kenneth Cooper at his Aerobics Center in Dallas. They followed 13,344 men and women for 15 years. This meticulous research, controlled for all major interfering variables, like age, family history, personal health history, smoking, blood pressure, cardiovascular condition, and insulin metabolism.

At the fifteen-year follow-up, reduced risk of death was closely correlated with physical fitness. This included death from cardiovascular diseases, a variety of cancers, and even accidents.

There is no longer any doubt: activity can save your life, while couch potatoism creates an existence that is nasty, sick, and short.

Activity Strengthens Heart and Lungs

Numerous studies show that exercise protects your body by maintaining vital capacity, and therefore maintaining adequate oxygenation of tissues.

The average sedentary American male aged 45 has lost half his ability to take up and use oxygen. With one year of the right exercise, he can restore it to the level of a 25 years old. Dr. Bortz rightly stated that the health benefits of restoring vital capacity are superior to any drug or medical treatment in existence.

In contrast to the weak cardiac function of sedentary folk, the athlete's strong, slow pulse is telling evidence of a healthy heart. Many have rates in the 40s, and the Colgan Institute one recorded champion cyclist Howard Doerfling at an incredible 29 beats per minute.

Sedentary folk, however, are likely to show heart rates in the 80s or 90s. When heart rate rises above 84, risk of coronary heart disease more than doubles.

Activity Protects Blood Pressure

The majority of average people show blood pressure of 120/80, which is regard as normal but this is not normal at all. We know now that these people are already on their way to disease. Risk of cardiovascular disease starts to rise as systolic blood pressure goes above 103 mmHg.

By 120 mmHg, previously thought to be normal, risk has risen from 51 to 77 per 10,000 people. That is an increase of 50 per cent.

By 135 mmHg, a level that many physicians still regard as marginal, but acceptable, risk has doubled. Beyond 135 mmHg you are a walking time bomb.

The same applies to diastolic blood pressure. Usual levels found in average people are 80-89 mmHg. Recent research show that these figures indicate a pre-disease state.

Diastolic pressures below 80 mmHg shows an incidence of new cardiovascular disease of 10 cases per 1000 people, but by 90-89 mmHg it shows an incidence of 40 cases per 1000 people, a risk increase of 300 per cent.

Don't fret. It's easy to reduce blood pressure with the right exercise.

Many studies show that exercise works for older people as well, in whom you might think the damage to blood pressure is permanent.

In a typical study, sedentary hypertension patients, aged 55 to 78 years were followed.

All had elevated blood pressure.

After participating in an exercise program, systolic blood pressure felt by a whopping 20 mmHg. Regular exercise will lower blood pressure in almost anyone.

Activity Lowers Cholesterol

Despite media bleating, cholesterol is not the bad guy.

Cholesterol is essential to every function of your body.

It forms part of all your organs, including your heart and your brain.

Your body makes all your steroid hormones, including adrenalin, estrogen and testosterone from cholesterol. You cannot live without it.

Most of your cholesterol is not from food at all. It is manufactured in your body mainly by the liver. When a healthy person eats high cholesterol foods, the liver immediately reduces its own cholesterol production to keep blood cholesterol low and healthy.

Disordered cholesterol metabolism is the cause that blood cholesterol rises to dangerous levels and is a man-made disease, caused mainly by our degraded nutrition and sedentary lifestyle.

As you probably know, we have "good" high-density lipoprotein (HDL) and "bad" low-density lipoprotein cholesterol. Total cholesterol is mostly LDL and this is still one of the best predictors of cardiovascular disease.

You can measure this total cholesterol with a simple device at home, it is called the "Accumeter".

What is a healthy cholesterol level? You may ask. The American Heart Association and other US health authorities made in mid-1980 below 200 mg/dl their official recommendation.

Today we know that this is too high. In a comprehensive study by Dr Jeremiah Stamler, he followed 356,000 men in 28 US cities. Following his research, death rates from cardiovascular disease starts to rise when cholesterol gets above 168 mg/dl.

Total cholesterol in sedentary American men and women rise over 200 mg/dl in their 30s and reach about 220 mg/dl by age 45.

It's clear that sitting like a slug expose oneself to disease. Recent research shows that average cholesterol levels in runners and bodybuilders ranged between 158 mg/dl and 183 mg/dl. It proves that exercise makes the healthy difference.

Cardiovascular diseases are far out our **biggest health problem.**

It kills more than twice as many Americans as all cancers, nine times as many as all other lung and liver diseases together, and 28 times more than all forms of diabetes.

There are good reasons to warn everybody starting an exercise program to have a thorough medical and physician's approval before they start.

Sudden exertion in sedentary people "raises their changes of a heart attack by….100 fold!

A health letter from the Mayo Clinic stated:

'Most people who have heart attacks during activity are sedentary or have underlying heart disease and overdo it.'

Activity Prevents Cancer

Most cancers are slow-growing diseases, eating silently away at your body for years before they show up.

Despite the overblown claims of successful treatment by the National Cancer Institute, once a cancer emerges, medicine is usually powerless.

Remember the swift deaths of Michael Landon of pancreatic cancer and Jaqueline Onassis of Lymphoma. If there was an effective treatment, don't you think those immensely rich people would have bought this?

So, if a little of the right exercise can prevent cancer, it's worth than all the gold in Ford Knox. And above all, like the other best things in life, it's free!

From a study by Dr. Kenneth Cooper, it showed that incidence of all forms of cancer was closely correlated with lack of physical exercise. Unfit men and women where 300 per cent more likely to develop cancer.

But the best finding from this study is that you have to move only a smidgen out of couch potato land to prevent cancer big time.

Activity: Protection against All Diseases

The right exercise is a major strategy for **protection against all diseases.**

Physicians who do not incorporate exercise into their treatment protocols are **guilty of malpractice.**

The right exercise maintains your heart, lungs, your muscles, your bones, a healthy level of bodyfat, even your intestinal function.

But what about more subtle functions, such as insulin, and your body's handling of sugar?

We know that couch potatoism leads to glucose intolerance.

However, research has shown not long ago that getting off the couch not only maintains insulin function to deal with the sugar, but also can reverse decades of damage. In healthy people the right exercise completely protects glucose tolerance against the degenerative changes in insulin metabolism that lead to adult-onset diabetes.

Research has revealed the major way in which **activity gives you protection against all diseases.** It started with evidence that exercise increases overall white blood cells.

Then came more precise findings that moderate exercise increases bodily production of **lymphocytes, interleukin 2, neutrophills**, and other disease fighting components of the immune system. There is no longer doubt that the right exercise strengthens your immunity. Remember the wise words of Louis Pasteur, the father of modern medicine: "Host resistance is the key".

Hence activity strengthens your resistance against all sorts of damage, decay, bacteria, viruses, toxins, even radiation and gives **protection against all diseases.** When we analyze the large number of health benefits which are responsible for physical fitness, it's easy to get motivated and get started with exercising, or to keep it up, whatever the case may be.

When we have health, we have hope, and when we have hope, we have everything!

29. The Truth About Exercise For Older Adults

Exercise is vital for any older adult who wants to remain healthy. Studies have shown that older adults who exercise regularly have better balance and a lower risk of falls. They have better control of their blood sugar levels, better flexibility, better quality of sleep and fewer symptoms of depression.

They will also improve their muscle strength and have less arthritis pain on their hips and knees.

There are many books and articles encouraging young and older people to exercise. It is easy to understand that exercise is good at any age, but to determine the right exercise program is not so easy, in fact, it can be difficult. People have different body shapes, different medical issues and different musculoskeletal problems.

That's the reason it is not advisable to start an exercise program that is not adjusted to meet the specific needs of the individual older adult. One has to carefully choose a trainer when joining a gym or health club. Many athletic trainers are not trained to understand all the potential risks and dangers involved with training the elderly.

The elderly person needs someone who understands the subtle issues that come with aging muscles and ligaments. In addition, many seniors have arthritis and osteoporosis, which changes the normal body alignment during exercise. Others may have degenerative changes in the spine. If a trainer doesn't pay attention to these details, the person could get hurt. You have to train a seventy-eight-year-old woman differently than an eighteen-year-old football player. You have to be very careful.

Aerobic Exercise

Endurance exercise will help you to strengthen your heart and lungs. It increases your stamina as well. Many older adults have much atherosclerosis (plaque) in their coronary arteries, which places them at a higher risk for heart attacks. For older adults who have not exercised for years should talk to their doctor first before starting an aerobic exercise program. The doctor may determine whether the person's heart is able to tolerate the increased exertion associated with exercise.

It is generally recommended that people should try to exercise for thirty minutes at 75 per cent to 80 per cent. of their maximum target heart rate. The maximum heart rate is calculated using the simple formula 220 - your age in years. This formula doesn't work well for many seniors. For the older adult who has not exercised for years and wants to start exercising, it is recommended to set a goal of 60 per cent – 65 per cent, rather than 75 – 80 per cent. For those who can't exercise for the full 30 minutes, two 15 minutes periods or three 10 minutes periods may suffice.

Be careful before you buy any of those heart rate meters, if you are on heart medications called beta-blockers, which can slow down their heart rate. Many pacemakers regulate how fast the heart can beat. If you have an irregular heart rhythm problem called atrial fibrillation, you also have to be careful. So how hard should elderly people exert themselves? It is suggested that they should be able to talk comfortably while exercising.

Stretching

With stretching exercises you also have to be careful, especially if you haven't stretched for decades. During that time your tendons (which attach muscles to bones) and ligaments (which attach bones together), have undergone a variety of degenerative changes and the water content decreases. The water content of cartilage also decreases. As a result, most people become less flexible as they age. Tendons and ligaments tend to tear easier and when they tear, the healing process is slower.

Here are some helpful hints on stretching from the National Institute on Aging: Stretching exercises should only be done after a warming up period by walking or some gentle bicycle riding. Especially during the wintertime when your joints and ligaments are stiffer because of the cold weather. Stretching should cause some minor discomfort, but it should not be painful. If you are getting pain, you need to lessen the tension or stop. Move slowly into a stretching position. Quick jerking motions can cause an injury. Hold the position for at least twenty to thirty seconds. If you can't hold the stretch that long, than you are overstretching and you need to do it more gently. We believe that all frail elderly people should consult with their physician or their physical therapist before starting a stretching regimen. Don't do just stretching exercises that you saw someone perform TV or at the gym. Even a yoga or Pilates class that is not specifically designed for the untrained older adult can lead to injuries.

Weight Training

There is some truth in the saying: "use it or lose it". The real truth is that many elderly folks don't have much more that they can afford to lose. This brings up the concept of functional reserve, which refers to the amount of extra work that can be done by an organ or muscle when needed. By the time some seniors reach their eighties or nineties, they have such a small functional reserve in their muscles that they can barely out of bed or walk.

Many seniors take up exercise programs that involve lifting weights. By lifting weights their muscles will grow in size and become stronger. Weight training would appear on the surface to make sense. Increasing muscle size and strength could help many seniors who have lost some of their size and strength over the years.

The real truth is that older adults need to be careful before beginning a weightlifting program. Proper instruction with the correct weight and form is critical. We cannot over emphasize the danger that a poorly designed weight training regimen poses to the joints, tendons and ligaments of seniors. Studies have shown that a carefully designed regimen may make seniors' muscles a little bigger and stronger. Any benefits gained have usually been lost once the study is over. Researchers have not been able to show that weight-training exercises by themselves can decrease the level of disability among frail seniors.

Some recommendations for folks who have not exercised for decades.

1. Walking - it is very simple and very effective. Even 15 minutes twice a day can help improve one's lung function and lowers the blood sugar levels in patients with diabetes. For people who are out of shape, this is a nice way to exercise without putting much stress on the joints.

2. Pool exercises - you don't have to do laps in the pool. Walking in the pool or simply moving your arms and legs as you stand in the shallow end of the pool is an excellent way to exercise. Buoyancy provides support to joints during movement and even provide some resistance. Muhammad Ali used to do pool exercises to help him train for many of his fights. It works very well for patients with arthritis of the hips and knees as a way to exercise arthritic joints without putting much weight-bearing stress on the joints.

3. Stationary bicycle - when done at low speeds and low resistance this exercise can be of great benefit for patients with arthritic knees.

4. Tai chi - this Chinese martial art promote balance and strengthening without putting much stress on the joints and ligaments. Although it does not involve punching or kicking, it is still considered a martial art. It has also been shown in several studies to improve balance and decrease the risk of falls in older adults.

5. Yoga - many older adults enroll in yoga classes to be able to enjoy its many health benefits. These benefits include increased flexibility, improved balance, and an improved sense of well-being. However, older adults must be very careful. There are yoga classes that cater for clients who have medical challenges as well as older adults. Look for a yoga instructor who has experience in adapting poses for individual needs.

6. Custom exercises - for patients who can no longer walk, there are even exercises that a physical therapist can design to be done in bed or in a chair.

It is recommended to start slowly with exercise. Once started, some folks get quite motivated and excited about their new exercise regimen. The improvement in how they feel and in their exercise performance helps to motivate them further. As the amount of exercise increases, we often see that many of them succumb to joints and ligament injuries. The point is that even if you think you can do more, it is advised not to do so.

Questions to ask your doctor

1. Is it save for me to exercise?
2. What type of exercise should I be doing?

3. Are there exercises I should avoid doing?

A final tip: Proceed with caution when starting an exercise program. Start easy and work your way up slowly.

30. Can High-Intensity Aerobics Reverse the Aging Process?

Mayo researchers compared high-intensity interval training, resistance training and combined training in a twelve-week study. They monitored molecular and metabolic changes in adults, divided into age groups of between 18 and 30 and between 65 and 80 years.

All kinds of training increase lean body mass and insulin sensitivity, but only high-intensity and combined training improves aerobic capacity and mitochondrial function in skeletal muscle.

Mitochondria are tiny energy-producing structures inside cells. They change with age and activity, and tend to decrease, both in content and function, as we grow older. One result is that we have less energy.

In the study, high-intensity interval training also improved muscle protein content that not only allowed cells to create more energy, but also caused muscles to grow bigger, especially in older adults.

The ability of the mitochondria to generate energy was increased by 69 per cent among the seniors, and by 49 per cent in the younger group.

You should make sure that your heart is exercised every day. Aerobic exercises stimulate the respiratory and circulatory systems. As a result, you will supply fresh oxygenated blood to your cells, and your body will function more efficiently.

The heart is like any other muscle, if you don't use it, you will lose it! Do something every day, preferably early morning for half an hour.

You can choose from many aerobic activities: swimming, tennis, skipping robe, light jogging, bike riding, stretching and brisk walking, as well as aerobic classes. If you don't have the time to go to the gym, you can probably buy some equipment to exercise at home, for example rebounding on mini trampolines. Rebounding is a terrific aerobic exercise for all ages, that you can do at home or even better, in the garden.

It strengthens and tones every cell of the body, because it works against the gravity pull. Your heart rate will slow down, which is important. The lower the better. Mine is at 60 beats/minute and has been like that for a long time.

Don't make the mistake of excluding exercise from your daily life. A walk in the forest or at the seashore will do wonders for your physical well-being and for your emotional and spiritual outlook.

Weight-bearing exercises have several advantages above aerobics. Weight training significantly increase cardiovascular capacity and endurance. Weightlifting is better than aerobics to lose belly fat. It also increases muscle mass, thereby providing a more plentiful supply of glutamine for your immunity.

Apply high intensity forms of exercise and full-body resistance training. Low intensity cardio exercise has no effect for removing visceral fat in particular. High intensity exercise such as interval training, sprints (bike sprints or running sprints), AND full-body weight training are very effective at helping to improve your body's ability to manage glucose and increases insulin sensitivity, a crucial step in removing visceral fat.

These types of high intensity exercise routines are also very effective at increasing your fat-burning hormones and creating a hormonal environment conducive to burning off abdominal fat.

Don't train with weights for more than one hour per workout. Your ability to gain lean mass, is limited by your hormone levels. After 45 minutes to one hour, hormone levels decline. You can force yourself to continue, but it doesn't do your body any good.

Use a wide variety of exercises. Restricted resistance exercises, especially on machines, stress only certain fibres of a muscle in certain positions. You need to get all the fibres in all positions. You have to move some weights if you want a long and healthy life.

"We encourage everyone to exercise regularly, but the take-home message for older adults that supervised high-intensity training is probably the best, because, both metabolically and at the molecular level, it produces the most benefits, says Dr. K. Sreekumar an Nair, a Mayo Clinic endocrinologist and senior researcher on the study.

Another intense exercise that combines both strength training and aerobics is 'loaded carries'. In this type of exercise you carry a weight, appropriate for your capacity and health status and you walk with it outdoors. Slowly and gradually you may increase the amount of weight you carry. This increases strength and aerobic capacity, and it even increases testosterone in men.

There are several variations you may explore, and many articles and videos are available on the Internet. Put your health and safety first and rest appropriately and avoid competitive partners. I have developed a high-intensity exercise plan that contains aerobics, weightlifting and nutrition for athletes.

31. Lean For A Lifetime

Our greatest health risk is overweight, but it's not complicated to become lean, if you know how your body works. You might have tried commercial weight-loss systems or fad diets, or bogus slimming aids, which only set you up to become fatter.

You can save yourself the cost of professional visits, psychological counseling or complex behavior therapy, as most of such intervention is detrimental.

The National Institute of Health expert panel on weight loss showed that behavior therapy and counseling get worse long-term results then people who are losing weight by themselves.

The amount of fat you carry around is not determined by your genes, but by what you do and what you eat. Recent scientific studies have shown that neither the number of fat cells nor their seize is genetically fixed, but body fat is dependent on lifestyle.

Your body has no internal reference for a permanent level of fat, only for a habitual level. When you remain at a particular fat level for a year or more, your body develops all the adipose cells, capillaries, enzyme counts, peripheral nerves, hormone levels and connective tissues to support it. It becomes to recognize that level of fat as self and will defend it vigorously.

That's called your fat point. Your body constantly monitors its fat point with hormonal messages, such as glycerol, which warns the brain to take defensive action if even the smallest quantity of fat is suddenly used for fuel. That is why usual forms of dieting can't possibly work.

By slowing metabolism, increasing fat storage and increasing appetite, your body's fat point defenses will defeat you every time. Then how can you treat it? Easy!

Reliable studies show that it takes years of overeating to grow fat. Bodyfat accumulate very slowly, an ounce or so per day, a pound every two or three weeks. In a year you are 20 lbs. over. In 3 - 4 years you gain 60 lbs. of flab.

As your body shifts its habitual fat point up very slowly, you must operate down the same way, very slowly. Otherwise, your body will cannibalize your muscle, excite your fat storage enzyme, and boost your appetite to ravenous.

It's important to reduce you total daily calories by no more than 20 per cent. That's 400 calories off a 2000 calorie diet. That's 2800 calories or 0.8 lbs. of fat per week.

Because of increases in body efficiency, you will not lose 0.8 lbs. of fat but only about half a pound. That's the most you can lose without triggering body defenses.

Step 1.: Lose no more than half-a-pound of fat per week.

Get your body composition measured once a month, including fat weight, lean weight, and body water. A newly available alternative to underwater weighing is the inexpensive skin-fold calipers for self-use at home. These calipers have a tension device on them to ensure you get the same pressure on the fat each time you measure, provided you take the measurements in exactly the same spot every time.

Step 2.: Measure your body fat once a month.

The calories you cut from your diet must be the right calories, importantly from all kinds of fat. Contrary to the calorie-counting strategies of much of the weight-loss industry, we know that fat calories are fatter. When excess carbohydrates or protein are eaten, the body makes complex metabolic adjustments to promote glycogen storage in muscle and increase the use of protein or sugar for fuel.

It also must use a lot of energy to convert these foods to body fat. Hence you must eat a bigger excess of carbs and protein than you do of fat before they end up on your hips. But when excess fat is eaten, metabolism remains unchanged. Virtually all the excess is promptly layered onto all the wrong places.

Now you know why calorie counting doesn't work. Numerous recent studies show that you put on much more body fat by eating fat than by eating the same number of calories from carbs or protein. Fat calories pack on more body fat than calories from any other food.

Step 3.: Eat a low, low-fat diet.

Look on the nutrition facts label when you buy food. Divide the total calories by the calories from fat. If the answer is less than 5, don't buy the food. In a diet of 2000 calories, that's a maximum of 400 fat calories.

Step 4: Don't eat foods that contains more than 20 per cent fat calories.

Many dieters think that they are on healthy, low-fat nutrition, when in fact they are mis lead by false food labeling. Many apparently dry foods like cookies, baked goods, crackers & chips are higher in fat than ice-cream. Even low-fat milk is really high fat.

How does low fat milk get away with its name? By jiggery-pokery lobbying power, the dairy industry got an exemption from the new labels. Nevertheless, an 8 oz glass of low-fat milk (2%) serves you a hefty one-third of its calories from fat.

Food industry lawyers have filed exemption claims for all kinds of foods. So if you want to avoid hidden fats, don't trust anything on food labels except the Nutrition Facts panel. That must be accurate if it's legal.

Especially beware of "reduced fat" products. Under the label law "reduced fat" means 25 per cent less fat than the original product. So, it goes with everything from reduced fat bologna, high can still be 60 per cent fat, to "light" and "lite" variants of foods, that have to be one-third less fat than the original but can still be 40 – 50 per cent fat.

Step 5: Trust only the Nutrition Facts panel on food labels.

Next, you should cut down on simple sugars. Chocolate cookies, candy and table sugar are obvious, but raw sugar, refined honey, corn syrup, fruit juice concentrate and date sugar are bad as well. Look out for fruit juices, orange juice contains more sugar than Coca Cola.

What's the reason that sugar increase body fat? Because quick absorption into your bloodstream causes an excess insulin burst from the pancreas. When it reaches the liver, excess insulin, which is toxic, is converted into neutral triglycerides. Triglycerides are exactly the form of fats that are stored in all your adipose cells.

Sugar not only causes excess calories that turn to fat, but it also causes the body to make even more fat from its own insulin. Replace as much as the simple sugars in your diet by complex carbohydrates, like whole-grain and vegetables.

Step 6. Cut down on sugar, eat complex carbohydrates instead.

If you think you can lose weight by skipping a meal, forget it. It wouldn't work because this results in bursts as soon as you eat again. The excess insulin that will be turned into fat will compensate for the skipped meal. If you want to lose fat, you have to fast for a longer period, at least 24 hours. It's important to keep your insulin output level steady for the whole day. For optimum fat loss, reduce the size of your meals and eat five small meals per day.

Step 7. Don't skip meals, eat five small meals per day.

Almost all popular diets are deficient in essential nutrients. Don't fall in the trap of eating only grapefruit, bananas, and milk or only salad. By doing so you become nutrient deficient, it increases your appetite and makes you fatter. Instead, eat a large variety of foods.

Step 8. Avoid all fad diets-`

Most of our foods has become deficient in many vitamins and minerals. As a result, your body turns up your appetite and makes you to eat more to supply the missing nutrients. You must eat far too many calories to make up for the missing vitamins in your diet. A single nutrient deficiency is enough to make you fat like a hog.

The best solution to this problem is to take a full range, high quality multi-vitamin supplement plus a multi-mineral supplement every day. They act as a regulator to your appetite and naturally curb your desire to eat.

Step 9. Take a high-quality multi-vitamin and multi-mineral supplement every day.

The US National Academy of Sciences believed that chromium was great for car bumpers, but useless for human nutrition, till Dr. Walter Mertz of the Human Nutrition Research center in Beltsville, MD. Showed that chromium is essential for your body to use insulin.

Now the latest RDA handbook recommends 50-200 mcg of chromium every day to maintain insulin metabolism. Because of the large number of diabetes, folk are well aware that insulin enables the body to deal with sugar. What they usually don't know is that insulin also controls fat and muscle. However, unfortunately nobody gets even the minimum recommended level of chromium in their degraded food. Studies show that 90% of the selected diets contain less than 50 mcg of chromium per day. The average chromium intake is only 29 mcg.

As a result, this poor nutrition causes your insulin metabolism to barely limp along and your body fat piles up.

Dr Gary Evans developed a new form of chromium: chromium picolinate. More than 20 studies show that it improves insulin metabolism, reduces bodyfat and increases muscle mass. Pigs who have similar insulin metabolism to men, when fed chromium picolinate, increased their lean mass by 7 per cent and reduced their body fat by 21 per cent. That's a much healthier animal.

Your daily multi-mineral supplement should contain 200 mcg of chromium picolinate.

For fat loss you should use an additional 200 – 600 mcg of CP per day, in conjunction with an exercise program. Don't use any other form of chromium. Hexavalent chromium or chromate for example, is highly toxic.

Step 10. Use a chromium picolinate supplement every day.

Dr. Leonard Starline and his colleagues from the Garvin Institute for Medical Research in Australia, were the first to prove that omega-3 fatty acid found in fish oils and also made by our body from Alpha-linolenic acid in flax oil, improve insulin efficiency, by using carbohydrates and fats for fuel.

Most Americans are deficient in omega-3s. It's important to get it to combat body fat.

Step 11. Take a flax oil essential fatty acid supplement every day.

The bodyfat stored in adipose cells is carried by a nutrient called l-carnitine, to the mitochondria (furnaces) of muscle cells, where it is burned for energy. By increasing the level of l-carnitine by means of supplementation, more bodyfat is transported and burned.

Your body makes l-carnitine, but if you are overweight and yet don't eat a lot, your body doesn't make enough for optimum use of fat for fuel. To improve fat loss, take 2-4 grams of l-carnitine per day in conjunction with exercise. Make sure you get l-carnitine, not racemic- or dl carnitine, which is cheap and toxic and interferes with l-carnitine metabolism and consequently increases body fat. Don't except cheap l-carnitine.

Step 12. Take an l-carnitine supplement every day.

Make sure to take 30 - 50 gram high-fiber per day to prevent disease and to create slow and even food absorption from your intestines, keeping your insulin level steady and also promote the use of food for energy rather than for the building up of body fat.

The average American don't get more than 10 - 20 gram of fiber per day, which promote a lot of diseases and put on body fat. Fiber is essential to prevent colon and rectal cancer.

Step 13. Eat 40 gram of mixed fibers per day.

Dr. Peter Wood from Stanford University has shown frequently that exercise is more important than food intake to keep body fat under control. As a regular exerciser you can eat a lot more and keep slimmer than sedentary people. If a plump person does the right exercise at the right time, he can increase his caloric intake far above the amount used by the exercise and still lose a lot of fat.

The key is to do the right exercise.

Aerobics are usually recommended in the weight loss industry, the more intense the better, which is all wrong!! The problem is that aerobics exercises that raise your heart rate above 120 beats per minute, which include running, rowing, swimming, cycling and many of those fancy aerobics classes in health clubs, all strip off muscle almost as much as they strip off fat.

And as you know, muscle loss reduces your ability to burn fat and sets you up to become even fatter. Remember, muscle is the engine in which body fat is burned. You should do everything you can to maintain it for the rest of your life.

Walking is good for many health reasons: it also burns some fat and will not burn muscle. But the best exercise for fat control is wide-variety high repetition resistance training, using weights or machines. By exercising all the muscles of your body, you burn a lot of fat.

Another advantage of resistance exercise is that it increases muscle and as a result provide more muscle cells to be able to burn fat. It's a real health bargain.

Step 14. Do high-repetition, wide-variety resistance exercise.

The basic rules for muscle work are simple. If you use heavy resistance so that you can complete only 3 - 6 repetitions of an exercise and you do 5 - 6 sets, you build maximum strength, but you don't lose much fat. If you reduce the weight so that you can complete 8 - 12 repetitions and you do 3 - 4 sets, you build muscle well and burn medium amounts of fat.

If you set the weight so you can run out of steam in 20 - 25 repetitions, while doing only one set, you build a little muscle but burn a lot of fat.

Step 15. For maximum fat-loss, do one set of each exercise with a weight that exhausts you in 20 - 25 repetitions.

It might be true that running burns more calories than walking and cross-country skiing burns most calories of all, but fat loss has little to do with calories used during an exercise session. Many recent studies show that the right exercise raises your metabolic rate for up to 18 hours afterwards. However, if you exercise in the evening and then go to bed, you lose most of the fat loss effect, because sleep causes your metabolism rate to drop rapidly. The best time to exercise is in the mornings, the earlier the better.

Step 16. Exercise in the mornings.

Dr. Leonard Epstein analyzed all the published studies on exercise and fat loss and showed that people who exercise five times per week lose three times as much fat as those who exercise only twice or three times per week, even if they exercise for a longer period. Those who exercise only once per week lost no fat at all.

For fat loss, five days weekly exercise of 30 minutes is much superior to three days weekly of 70 minutes, even though the total weekly exercise time of the three-day people is an hour longer. In order to keep that metabolic rate churning, frequent exercise is the key.

Step 17. Exercise five mornings weekly for a minimum of 30 minutes.

As you can read in my article about exercise, oxidation is the primary cause of human degeneration.

Because exercise uses 12 - 20 times more oxygen than sitting in a chair, it also creates masses of free radicals that causes a lot of oxidation damage. Without additional antioxidants you are slowly killing yourself. You can prevent exercise oxidation damage by taking antioxidant supplements.

Step 18. Take a multiple antioxidant every day.

The first strategy in your fight against body fat is to reduce your appetite. Phenylpropanolamine helps a little. Better is ephedrine hydrochloride and its original source: Ma Huang or Ephedra sinical. But you should be very sensible in the use of these compounds.

Don't use more than 25 - 50 milligram per day, otherwise it loses its effect and can cause many side-effects, including raised blood pressure, anxiety, and insomnia.

The second strategy is to reduce the taste of food, especially sweet tastes. The herb Genoa Silvestre has been used for this purpose for thousands of years in Ayurvedic medicine. It works a bit.

The third strategy is to reduce your body's tendency to store fat. The herb Garcinia cambogia, a specific variant of the English brindleberry is used in Ayurvedic medicine for this purpose. The active ingredient is hydroxy citrate.

Ongoing studies by DR. Andrew Weil at the University of Arizona indicate that 500 milligrams of garcinia may reduce fat storage from a high-fat meal by up to 30%. As a bonus, it may also reduce appetite.

The final strategy is to raise metabolic rate so that your body burns more calories during the day. It's called thermogenesis, which means it raises body temperature. To maintain the increased temperature, the body must burn more calories to make the heat - lots of calories. And because it is low level activation, the calories burned come mainly from fat.

There are a lot of drugs that does the job, but all of them causes side effects. It doesn't make sense to make yourself unhealthy while trying to lose fat. Least damaging are the beta-adrenergic agonists and most harmless of these is ephedrine or its herbal source: Ma huang. These compounds work by increasing bodily output of noradrenalin, one of our "fight-or-flight" hormones.

That warns you right away not to use too much (25-50 mg per day max.) or you run into severe anxiety, irritability, headache and insomnia. The FDA are against ephedrine, because folk have used larger doses and caused real damage to the thyroid gland and other organs.

However, ephedrine on its own is not effective, because your body quickly defends itself with multiple mechanisms that turn off the extra noradrenalin. The three main defenses your body uses against a sensible ephedrine regimen (25--50 milligram/day) are: increasing output of phosphodiesterase enzymes, and increasing prostaglandin production. These defenses can be overcome respectively by using caffeine, theophylline (from tea) and acetylsalicylic acid (aspirin). Herbal sources can also supply the caffeine, theophylline and aspirin.

Standardized extracts of kola nut, guarana, black tea and white willow are good sources. And you can prolong the effect of caffeine, which is mildly thermogenic by itself, by using naringenin, a compound found in grapefruit.

Another effective chemical to use in conjunction with beta-receptor agonists is yohimbine, a compound from the bark of the yohimbe tree. Yohimbe is one of the class of compounds called selective antagonists of alpha-2 receptors. This action of yohimbine has shown to cause long- term thermogenesis and fat loss in animals.

Controlling excess body water is the last thing you can do to lose body fat. Especially for women, who have this problem. Bloating and edema prevent your Lean For Life program, because they make you feel blah and make you to sit like a slug and avoid exercise.

Diuretic drugs are not the solution, but mildly diuretic foods like melons, cucumber, grapes, apples, parsley, pineapple and cooked asparagus all help to shed excess water. Mil diuretic herbs, like Uva ursi and Sarsaparilla also have a use in this phase of fat loss.

Step 19. Use the right herbal fat loss supplement every day.

Success is always achieved by setting goals. To improve your performance, you should set specific goals and sub-goals and write them down and post them on the fridge, for example, so that everybody can see them.

Goals must be specific, measurable and time limited. "To lose weight" is too vague. Instead for example: to lose 10 lbs. of fat by my next birthday is a good goal.

Lean for Life is a very long-term goal, so you must use sub-goals to be able to check your progress.

Finally, you have to make your goals public, so that your family and friends can blame you for failure, but praise & reward you for success.

Step 20. Form specific, measurable, public, rewarded fat loss goals.

Diet And Fitness

If you are looking for some practical advice that will enable you to lose weight and keep it off permanently, the following information will help you with this.

For fat loss, five days weekly exercise of 30 minutes is much superior to three days weekly of 70 minutes, even though the total weekly exercise time of the three-day people is an hour longer. To keep that metabolic rate churning, frequent exercise is the key.

Depriving yourself is not the answer to healthy, permanent weight-loss. Deprivation and bingeing become a vicious circle, and that's just one of the many problems with dieting.

Another thing is that diets are temporary, therefore, the results must be temporary. The fact of the matter is that dieting does not work. It never has and it never will. If diets worked, would the rate of obesity in America not decreasing each year instead of increasing? In 1982, fifteen billion dollars were spent on weight-loss schemes in the USA alone! If diets worked, that incredibly high amount of money would surely put an end to this problem, wouldn't it? The fact is, that this ridiculous high amount is increasing by one billion dollar every year. In spite of the new diets that come and go, the problem is becoming worse.

However, no weight loss program nor the benefits mentioned in this article will work without proper exercise.

Overweight Is Illness

According to the Framingham Heart Study, America's best, shows that weight gain after adulthood causes a huge risk increase of all type of cardiovascular disease. Even a 10% increase above ideal weight causes a 6-7per cent increase in blood pressure. Losing that extra weight causes an immediate drop in blood pressure of 10-11 per cent.

Women, carrying 50-60 lbs. of extra weight are 700% more likely to develop hypertension. Both men and women carrying 60 lbs. extra or more have a 3000% more change of developing diabetes.

The results of a 20-year study by the American Cancer Society, involving over 1 million Americans in 25 different states showed that men who are 40% overweight, have higher rates of prostate cancer, colon cancer and rectal cancer.

Women who are 40% overweight, have higher rates of breast cancer, ovarian cancer, uterine cancer, gall bladder cancer, cervical cancer and endometrial cancer. Corpulent is sick indeed!

Overweight is a significant cause of almost all diseases. Even moderate fatness damages the immune system and reduce your resistance to everything. Overweight people going into surgery increase their risk of post-operation infections by up to 700%. Studies show that fat babies get twice as many infections as slim babies.

Moderately overweight folk show typical defensive reactions to the evidence that fat is sick. They suck in their stomachs and laughing proclaim: "This is just happy fat." Or they slap their plump thigh and exclaim: "God made me this way, healthy and comfortable."

The latest study at the Harvest School of Public Health shows that even the mildly chunky die young. Dr. I-min Lee tracked 19,297 healthy Harvard men who graduated between 1916 and 1950. Smokers were excluded as unacceptable health risks.

By 1988, 4370 of the men had died, mostly chunky. The less the men weighted, the lower their death risk. Men who were 20% below the average had the best change for a long and healthy life.

Body fat is by far America's worst health risk, with 32.6 million Americans classified as overweight and about 40 million on the way. It causes more illness than all the environmental and nutrition problems, than smoking, alcohol and all other drugs put together. It's infinitely worse than over-publicized AIDS.

Yet, to the ignorant, overweight is little more than a good butt for humor. It is sort of comical, that Americans waddle enough fat around to feed the whole of starving Africa and would gladly pay the shipping, but the disease it causes is no joke.

The industry around weight loss is well aware of the fact that low-calorie diets cause fast loss of muscle and fat. For this reason, the market is saturated with fiber bars, liquid meals and light weight cereals.

We live in a society of instant coffee,….. while-you-wait, etc. Fast results are essential for continuous sales results. The average consumer is not aware of the fact, that when they are losing fat, they lose muscle also.

Nutrition scientists have known for many years that reducing calories to 800 – 1200 per day, which is below the essential energy requirement of the body to maintain vital functions, causes you to cannibalize your own muscles for fuel. On these diets, muscle provides up to 45% of the energy deficit.

If the deficit in essential energy requirement is 500 calories per day, then up to 225 calories will come from muscle breakdown. On only four weeks on such a diet, you can lose 1.5 kg of vital muscle. In your muscles is all your energy created by burning of fats, carbohydrates, and proteins in the mitochondria of every cell.

Even an ounce of muscle lost, lowers basic metabolic rate of fuel consumption and reduces your ability to burn body fat.

So, all diets that are below the essential energy requirement of your body are a guaranteed recipe for failure.

Besides the fact of losing muscle, which is your body's engine, the weight loss industry also know that fast fat loss guaranties regain of fat. The physiology behind it has been known for decades.

Fast fat loss alerts the potent defense of the body of its energy reserve. The quantity and activity of the lipo protein lipase enzyme increases immediately, which is the body's main mechanism that collect digested fat from the bloodstream and stuff it into fat cells.

Lipo protein lipase gets hold of every fat molecule and even disable your body to use it for energy. In order to make up the deficit, you have to burn more muscle. However, as muscle is your basic structure, it is harder for your body to burn it than fat. As a result, your metabolism slows down, which reduces your ability to burn fat.

Toxic wastes build-up as a result of burning proteins. This can make you sick and cranky. This activity does not help you to control your appetite, which becomes more ravenous.

It gets even worse. If you can't resist the inconvenience any longer and succumb to real food, the lipo protein lipase has become so efficient, that you regain seven weeks painful fat loss in almost seven days.

But the biggest problem is that you don't get any of the lost muscle back.

So, the final result of the diet is that there is no change in body fat but a big loss in muscle. This loss of part of your engine causes further fat gain as it reduces your ability to burn the fat you have.

Overweight people using low-calorie diets lose so much muscle that they set their bodies up for permanent obesity, when they use them repeatedly.

The food industry is constantly creating new 'functional foods' that will help you lose weight, reduce blood pressure and cholesterol, and help you keep your blood sugar and insulin levels in check and so on and so on.

When did eating become so complicated, and since when could food do all of these magical things?

Foods designed to help you lose weight are a multi-billion-dollar industry.

And think of how ironic of an industry that is, how could you possibly eat something to lose weight? That doesn't make any sense at all. The act of eating always adds mass to your body, it couldn't possibly take it away.

The only way you can lose weight ever, is to eat less calories than you burn off. Bottom line, there is no arguing this.

This rule existed 1000 years ago and will exist 1000 years from now. There is no possible way you could gain weight if you ate less calories than you burned off. No matter how easy you seem to put on weight, and how little food you think you eat, there is always a lesser amount that will cause you to lose weight.

The actual matter that makes up your fat cells must come from somewhere, and that somewhere is your diet. If you eat more food than you burn off then you will store fat and gain weight. If you eat less food than you burn off you will lose fat and lose weight. That's it.

So, the list of 7 foods you can eat to lose weight consists of any foods you would like to see on that list! You could lose weight eating cheesecake every day. As long as you ate fewer total calories that day than you burned off.

The only weight loss diets that have ever worked or proven to have any effect always make people eat fewer total calories. That's it. Carbohydrate, fat, protein, and sugar don't make any difference, as long as you eat less. If anyone tells you otherwise, they just haven't done their research. And I encourage you to challenge anyone who thinks that any 'special' food can actually help you lose weight. It's baloney, eating less is the only way. Think of it this way. If any of the popular diets like low carbohydrate, low fat, high protein actually worked, would you or anyone else still be looking for another way to lose weight?

There are three main keys to losing fat and gaining muscle. If you're missing any of these, you will most likely fail in your attempts to build a lean muscular body.

So, what are they?

1) Eat Less Calories than you burn off

2) Resistance Training

3) Eating enough protein to maintain muscle mass

That's as short and sweet as I can put it. Any diet can work as long as it gets you to eat less calories than you burn off. The key is to find a diet that suits your personality and your lifestyle.

If you're like me you don't have time to spend on diet rules and focusing on good foods and bad foods and what to eat and what not to eat, and meal timing and all of that.

The diet that will work for you will most likely be the one with the least amounts of rules, or in fact no rules at all but rather just provide a guideline or two.

For me that diet is Eat Stop Eat.

It is the simplest nutrition program I have ever come across. There is only one guideline, and that is to take a 24-hours break from eating once or twice per week. That's it, simple and effective. This type of eating program might work for you, or it might not.

You just must try it first. As long as you can find a diet you can stick with for the long term, you'll be able to lose weight, the next key is making sure all of that weight comes from fat.

This is where resistance training comes in. You must do some form of resistance training in order to maintain and build muscle mass while you're losing fat. If you are following an effective diet without doing resistance training you could end up losing muscle mass along the way. If this happens you could lose body weight without actually improving the look or shape of your body.

Your actual body weight doesn't matter as much as your percentage of fat. If you can lose 5 pounds of fat but gain 3 pounds of muscle you will only lose 2 pounds of body weight on the scale, but you'll look 8 pounds different. Even though 2 pounds doesn't sound like much, the difference on your body fat percentage is the key.

This is why weight training is so important while dieting. Weight training is the best way to make sure you don't lose muscle while you diet, this helps with overall health as well as improving the overall look and shape of your body.

After all, when you diet the goal is to show off the lean muscle that is under the fat. You build a great body in the gym and in the kitchen and which is more important will vary from person to person. Is there something about exercise that make some people hungrier than they were before?

In fact, there is. Exercise, by definition, is problematic. When researchers have used exercise as a short – or long-term intervention to help people to lose weight, it doesn't work the way it's supposed to. Average weight-loss in exercise-only studies is often minuscule.

The third key to building muscle while losing fat is protein. You have to eat just enough protein to make sure your muscles can grow. This is a controversial topic that many nutrition 'experts' still don't agree on. But the bottom line is protein is your friend when it comes to building muscle and especially when you're dieting.

Mix these three key ingredients together and you'll have a potent fat loss and muscle building program that can transform your body in no time.

32. Chemicals In Our Environment

Hundreds of thousands artificial chemicals have been unleashed, of which approximately 75,000 are in common use around the world, with more than 3,500 used in food processing. Every year, half a billion kg of pesticide are deposited into the environment.

The pesticide contamination is so widespread that DDT residues are found in penguins at the South Pole, thousands of kilo meters from where the pesticide was applied, and its metabolites have been found in most of the samples of human and animal tissues ever tested.

Toxic chemicals have been found in wild animals, in the oceans, in our drinking water, in our homes, in soils and in women's breast milk.

"It has been almost impossible for governments to control this industrial bonanza and we are now living in a world without meaningful controls **over toxic chemicals," according to** Eve Hillary, author of "Children of a toxic harvest." Nor do we have much idea about the combined effects (Synergy) of the different chemicals. In which the combination may be far more toxic than any of the originals alone.

When we consider that most of these chemicals accumulate in our fatty tissues and that the brain is high in fat, the potential for harm from prolonged exposure is very high.

Although nobody can avoid some degree of contamination, a lot of **unnecessa**ry use of chemicals can be avoided. Minimizing exposure to chemicals can make the difference between health and a nightmare of difficult to **explain symptoms.**

When we avoid the chemicals that we can avoid, our bodies are probably be able to cope with the chemicals, we can't avoid. We need to exercise as much care as we possibly can to avoid coming into daily contact with the chemicals that are forced upon us.

Man-made, synthetic or artificial chemicals are technically called xenobiotic, this means they are foreign to life. They effect the energy production of every cell in our body and thereby effecting every system, in particular our immune system.

The consequences may be allergies chronic fatigue syndrome, multiple chemical sensitivities, infertility, birth defect, artery disease, **stroke, cancer** and other conditions.

In general, toxic chemicals produce free radicals, highly destructive molecules, which cause tissue damage and eventually result in above mentioned degenerative diseases.

There is now evidence from a Danish study that the overall intelligence of school children is decreasing.

It is no surprise that the increasing number of chemicals cause a decline in the general health of populations around the world. One in three **Australians get ca**ncer during their lifetime and one in four die from it.

According to a 1994 Work safe Australia study, out of 2,700 deaths in Australia each year from work related causes, about 2,200 death **are the results of cancers caused by chemical exposure at work.**

33. How To Avoid Chemicals At Home

We are constantly warned by commercials that our homes are full of dangerous germs, and they must be killed, resulting in the addition of antiseptics in cleaning products. But they can be more harmful than most of the germs they kill.

Cleaning products with the most fumes are generally the most harmful, such as multi-purpose cleaners, disinfectants, and oven cleaners.

Use the proven safer cleaners, like pure soap or soap flakes for washing dishes and clothes, or use environmentally friendly cleansers like Planet Ark, Nutrimetics, GNLD, Herbon or Tri Nature.

For cleaning windows, tubs and tiles, try vinegar and water. For refrigerators, freezers, stainless steel, enamel, chrome and laminex, use bicarb soda.

Solvents

These chemical products are used to dissolve other substances.

Many solvents can cause health problems, like brain damage, birth defects, miscarriage, asthma and cancer. Long term exposure can cause progressive loss of memory and affect learning ability and decision making.

Some people with multiple chemical sensitivity and/or chronic fatigue syndrome are affected badly by solvents.

A study at Queen Elizabeth Hospital in Adelaide found a connection between solvents and miscarriage. In fact, the study found that miscarriage is four times more likely if the woman has been involved in home renovation or has visited factories with high chemical pollution and 2 to 3 times more likely if the male partner has been exposed to strong glues, oven cleaners or oil-based paints.

Solvents are present in many household products, including cleaning products, pesticides, liquid paper, marker pens, glues, and paints.

Out gassing of volatile organic compounds.

Paints, plastics, and particle boards in our homes can give off traces of toxic gasses for months and even years. This out gassing is worse in winter when heating is on, and windows are shut.

VOC's out gas from large surface areas, painted walls, ceilings, and stained floors. Also, from glued carpets, vinyl, shelves, furniture, particle boards and plastics.

Make sure that the house is always well ventilated and use paints and varnishes that don't out gas.

For floors use timber, tile, and linoleum that out gas very little.

Buy solid timber furniture.

Avoid sources of formaldehyde gas, a potent irritant that affects the respiratory system and can cause asthma. It evaporates from the glue in particle board, plywood, synthetic carpets, upholstery and sometimes wallpaper and some paints.

Non-Fluid Combustion Heating

When a gas, kerosene o wood heater doesn't have a chimney, it's called non fluid. It results in pollution that is often far worse than outdoors pollution.

The toxic fumes from these heaters can cause symptoms like throat infections and worsen sinus problems and asthma.

Reduce heating needs by dressing warmly and sleep with warm bedding (electric blanket).

Use electrical or fluid combustion heating and leave off when not required. Even better, design your house for solar heating.

Insulate the home with wool, cellulose or polyester. If non fluid combustion heaters must be used, make sure of adequate ventilation.

Dry-Cleaning Clothing

Dry-cleaning uses powerful solvents, like perchloroethylene, an organochlorine, which in extreme cases can damage the liver, kidneys and central nervous system.

After bringing home clothes from the dry cleaner, leave them outside, preferable in the sun for at least 24 hours. Avoid synthetic clothing and wear natural fibers like wool, cotton, linen, silk and mohair.

Fiberglass Insulation

Fiberglass can cause lung cancer in humans. Fibers with diameters of less than 3 microns can reach the tiny air sacs in the lungs and remain there indefinitely, with the risk of a form of cancer similar to that caused by asbestos.

Every few years check the condition of the fiberglass. Seek professional advice if the fiberglass crumbles to 'powder'.

Lead Exposure

Lead is a heavy metal that can cause brain damage, especially in children and during pregnancy. The more common low-level poisoning can cause learning difficulties, hyperactivity, and less immunity to infections. To avoid lead exposure, live well away from motor vehicle pollution, if possible. Take off shoes if there is flaking old paint to avoid bringing lead dust into the house. A hard floor is better than carpet.

Use a safe chemical stripper that emits fewer toxic fumes. Have blood tests, especially for children, if you live near main roads and if your home has flaking old paint.

Industrial Chemicals

Factories that manufacture or use toxic chemicals have the greatest risk of exposure. What is known about the toxic effect has been discovered by studying their effects on workers in such factories.

Avoid working in any industry that uses toxic chemicals.

Ensure adequate ventilation when toxic chemicals are present – even for photocopiers and laser printers in offices.

We can make a difference by our everyday lifestyle choices, because what we buy invents the future.

If we care about our personal health and the kind of planet we are handing over to our children and grandchildren, it is worth to contemplate about the things we purchase to create the type of world we like to live in.

For example, if more people bought organic grown food, it would become cheaper and the need for pesticides could be reduced.

It would be good to join a group of people, for example a multilevel marketing company or a lobby group which has the vision for a healthier and happier future.

34. Problems Concerning the Heart

The heart is a simple organ, who's main function is to pump blood throughout the entire body.

Congestive heart failure and cardiomyopathy are diseases of the heart muscle and can have several causes, like: hypertension, repeated or severe heart attacks, viral infections and infiltrative heart diseases like lupus or scleroderma.

In each case the disease weakens the heart muscle and disable it to handle the amount of blood it receives from the body. The heart tries to compensate for its weakened state by dilating and beating faster. Ultimately, blood backs up into the lungs, filling them with fluid.

This is called congestive heart failure. The patient starts to drawn on his or her own fluid. Weakening of the heart is called cardiomyopathy and is a very severe case of congestive heart failure, characterized by a large dilated heart.

When the heart muscle is weakened, it places an increased demand on the nutrients the heart cell need, in order to create energy. Because of excessive use of these nutrients, the heart muscle becomes depleted of CoQ10, which is the most important nutrient for energy creation.

Patients who take this supplement be able to replenish their weakened heart muscle's stores of CoQ10, generating more energy and compensate for its weakened state.

Patients should continue to supplement their traditional medical treatment over a long period of time.

Clinical studies on CoQ10, which involved 2,660 patients with heart failure, resulted in nearly 80 per cent improvement in three major symptom categories. CoQ10 can be a significant helpful supplement for the treatment of the heart muscle. Coenzyme Q10 (CoQ10) is a fat – soluble vitamin and a strong antioxidant. Coenzymes are cofactors, essential for a large number of enzymatic reactions within the body. CoQ10 is the cofactor for at least three very important enzymes, used within the mitochondria, which is the furnace of the cell, where its energy is produced.

Mitochondria enzymes are needed for the production of the high – energy phosphate and adenosine triphosphate, upon which all cellular functions depend. It is in the mitochondria where the energy starts, but where also dangerous by-products, free radicals, are created.

CoQ10 is very important to help neutralize free radicals and most importantly, to create energy. CoQ10 is produced by the body, but this is a complicated process. It is also found in a variety of foods, like organic meats, beef, sardines, mackerel, and peanuts.

Doctors need to learn and understand how natural products can help their patients. By supporting the natural function of the body and trying to enhance its ability to perform at optimal level; only then everything possible is done to benefit the healing process of the body.

35. How to Overcome Menopausal Problems

Menopause can be a time of great exuberance for many women. To feel a sudden sense of freedom is natural with concerns about pregnancy, unfettered by monthly periods, or the anxiety of starting a career, As though the rest of your life is truly your own.

Anthropologist Margaret Mead, who did some of her most exciting work when she was well past her fifties, says: "There is no more creative force in the world than the menopausal woman with zest,".

Nevertheless, the body does undergo some physical changes during menopause that can take the zest out of the best. Some of the symptoms many women experience around this time are hot flashes, mood swings, and insomnia. Many women (and their doctors) assumed for years that the discomfort of menopause was an inevitable part of the process. But it doesn't have to be that way. Many of the problems of menopause can be controlled or even eliminated by eating the right foods, says Isaac Schiff, MD. Chief of obstetrics and gynaecology at Massachusetts General Hospital in Boston and author of Menopause.

Diet is more important than ever now that many women worry about the risk of treating their menopausal symptoms with hormone replacement therapy (HRT).

Shifts of hormonal production as a woman approaches menopause, her ovaries begin to produce less of the female hormones estrogen and progesterone. At some point, the production of these hormones starts to be so little that menstrual periods stop, and the physical problems, such as hot flashes and mood swings begin.

Some of the long-term changes in the body caused by low hormone levels, are even more serious. Estrogen, for example, regulates a woman's cholesterol levels. When estrogen production goes down, cholesterol rises. Which causes many women to have the risk of heart disease, after they have passed menopause. Estrogen also plays a role in keeping a woman's bones full of calcium. When estrogen levels drop, the bones lose calcium at a very fast rate. Unless women take care to get extra calcium in their diets, their bones become thin and weak, a condition called osteoporosis.

"Getting enough calcium before, during and after menopause is one of the most important things a woman can do to prevent possibly disastrous bone fractures", says Dr Utian.

Here soy foods can make a difference, because there is some evidence that the phytoestrogens in soy play an active role in helping bones keep their calcium. Holding on to calcium is important because many women don't get anywhere near enough of this important mineral. on average, women between ages 20 and 50 get about 600 milligram per day, and women past menopause get only about 500 milligram per day.

Scientist at the National Institutes of Health recommend that women in their childbearing years get at least 1000 milligram of calcium per day. Women past menopause should aim for 1,500 milligram per day.

Most women can get plenty of calcium from their diets. For example, 1 cup of fat-free milk contains 302 milligram of calcium, or 30 per cent of the Daily Value (DV). An 8-ounce serving of yogurt has 415 milligram or 41per cent of the DV, and 3 ounces of salmon has 181 milligram, or 18 per cent of the DV.

For years, many women replaced their estrogen levels with synthetic hormones, thinking it was a cure for everything, from hot flashes to high cholesterol. But in 2002, new research found that the hormones may actually increase the risk of heart disease, which led the National Institutes of Health and the American Heart Association to advice women not to take HRT to lower cholesterol or prevent a heart attack.

According to the Nurses' Health Study, postmenopausal women who have had a heart attack or have been diagnosed with heart disease and have been on HRT for less than a year have a 25 per cent higher risk of another heart attack or dying from heart disease than similar women who never have been on hormone therapy.

Although HRT still has advantages, such as protecting bones and easing problems in menopause, many women are looking for alternatives, and they're finding them in their own kitchens. Even women who do take HRT may find that making small adjustments to their diet will give them additional relief.

Protection from Soy Food Since many of the problems of menopause are caused by low levels of estrogen, it makes sense that replacing some of the estrogen will make women healthier. Scientists have found that certain foods – most importantly, soy foods such as tofu and tempeh – contain large amounts of phytoestrogens, plant compounds that act very much like the natural hormone.

In Asian countries, where women eat a lot of soy foods, only about 16 per cent have problems with menopausal discomfort. In fact, there isn't even a word in Japanese for 'hot flash'.

'Of course, it's always better to reach for the food, rather than the supplement', says Mary Jane Minkin, MD, clinical professor of obstetrics and gynecology at Yale University School of Medicine and author of A Woman's Guide to Menopause and Perimenopause. Dr Minkin recommends getting two servings of soy a day, such as a glass of soy milk and a serving of tofu. Or you could have a bowl of miso soup, which is flavoured with a condiment made from soybeans and salt.

Soy is also very important for protecting the heart, since a woman's risk for heart disease rises after menopause. Research has shown that eating more soy foods can help bring down cholesterol levels and the risk for heart disease.

Of course, when you're eating more soy foods, you're automatically eating less saturated fat, and this can also help keep cholesterol levels down. "Women approaching menopause and those who are already menopausal, should concentrate on having the heart-healthiest diet," adds Wulf H. Utian, MD, PhD, chairman of the department of reproductive biology at Case Western Reserve University in Cleveland. "It's one of the most important issues they face because of menopause."

For an alternative to soybeans, you can try eating black beans to reduce your hot flashes. They contain about the same number of phytoestrogens, and they can be cooked into great-tasting soups or sprinkled into salads.

Feel better with Flaxseed In addition to soy, it's a good idea to add flaxseed to your diet, Dr. Minkin says. Flaxseed is also a phytoestrogen that help relief hot flashes and sleep problems, the two complains Dr. Mirkin hears the most often from her patients going through menopause. Flaxseed also contains a large amount of lignans that may have antioxidant properties. which means they'll help menopausal women fight cancer. Of all the plant foods that contain lignans, flaxseed contains the most, at least 75 times more than other foods.

Add a tablespoon of ground flaxseed to your cereal or on top of your salad or bake it into bread or muffins. You don't need a lot of flaxseeds to get the benefits, Dr Minkin add.

Herbal Relief

Dr Minkin has found that taking 20 mg of the herb black cohosh helps her patients with menopausal problems. Because the United States doesn't regulate herbal products, she recommends buying the German brand Remifemin. Herbal products are regulated in Germany, and you'll know that you're actually getting what's on the label.

While the jury is still out on whether or not black cohosh is an effective treatment for menopausal symptoms, it wouldn't hurt to try the herb and see if it works for you.

Turn down the Heat There are some classic triggers for hot flashes. Here's how to avoid them and stay cool. Pass on hot foods. When it comes to temperatures and spiciness, hot foods are likely to bring on a hot flash, Dr Minkin says. It's a good idea to avoid hot beverages like hot soup or coffee. The same goes for spicy foods, such as Chinese or Mexican food.

Avoid red wine If you're going to drink, keep in mind that red wine is a classic trigger of hot flashes, says Dr Minkin. White wine isn't as bad, so it may be a better choice.

Dress for indulgences. If you really want to indulge in a spicy meal or drink a glass of red wine, prepare for a hot flash by dressing in layers. Wear a cardigan over something light so you can take off the top layer and cool off, Dr Minkin suggests. If you're at a restaurant, you may look for a table near a cool air vent or ask to sit away from the hot kitchen.

Doctor's Advice Menopausal symptoms such as hot flashes and sleep problems are certainly bothersome, but they're small potatoes compared with the higher risk of breast cancer and cardiovascular disease menopausal women face, says Jay Kenney PhD. RD, director of nutrition research and educator at the Prilikin Longevity Centre and Spa in Aventura, Florida.

Luckily, doing all of the things that protect you from cancer and heart disease will also help with your menopausal symptoms, so add some soybeans to your diet, and eat more whole grains, fruits and vegetables, and legumes. "The more the merrier," he says. "You can certainly eat beans every day. Have chili one day, black beans soup the next, a salad with garbanzo beans the next.

36. Prevention Of Memory Problems

Many researchers have discovered that when people are low in certain nutrients, their mental performance drops. Many people are fine as long as they meet their nutritional needs. Even not getting enough water can cause the mind to get fuzzy. The thirst mechanism slows down as we get older, as a result, we're not always aware right away that we need water. However, not all memory problems are caused by your diet, but when nothing else is wrong it may be what you eat that is slowing you down.

Vitamin B for the Brain The vitamin B complex are probably the most essential nutrients to keep your mind sharp. Your body needs the B vitamins to transform food into mental energy and to manufacture and repair brain tissue. "Deficiencies in thiamin, niacin and vitamin B6 and B12 can all cause mental dysfunction", says Vernon Mark, MD, author of Reversing Memory Loss. In fact, pellagra, a niacin deficiency, used to be a leading cause of admissions into mental hospitals," he explains. Research has shown that when children are given 5 mg thiamin instead of the Daily Value of 1.5 mg, they achieve remarkable higher scores when they are given tests of mental functioning, Dr. Mark adds.

Today, many cereals, breads and pastas are enriched with thiamin and niacin, so that most people are getting enough of these vitamins. Niacin deficiencies have become extremely rare, especially in this country. But in older people or those who frequently drink alcohol, levels of thiamin can drop low enough to cause memory problems, says Dr Mark.

The easiest way to make sure you get enough brain-boosting B vitamins is to eat foods that contain enriched grains. One cup of enriched spaghetti, for example, has 0.3 mg of thiamin, or 20 per cent of the Daily Value (DV), and 2 milligram of niacin, or 10 per cent of the DV. Meat is also a good source for getting these nutrients. Three ounces of pork tenderloin, for example, provide 0.8 milligram of thiamin, 53 per cent of the DV, while 3 ounces of chicken breast deliver 12 milligram or 60 per cent of the DV for niacin.

As we get older, it's not so easy to get additional amounts of vitamin B6 and B12, because it's harder for the body to absorb them. After the age of 55, it's common to be low in these vitamins, because the lining of the stomach is changing. When you get older, it's a good idea to get more than the DV of both of these nutrients. Vitamin B6 is abundant in baked potatoes, bananas, chickpeas, and turkey. One baked potato provides 0.4 milligram of vitamin B6, 20 per cent of the DV. and one banana provide 0.7 milligram or 35 per cent of the DV. For vitamin B12, meat and shellfish are good choices.

Maintaining the flow to the brain in order to avoid memory problems there should be sufficient blood flow to the brain. When adequate blood flow is not maintained, the brain and memory begin to perform poorly. The lack of blood to the brain is often caused by the same problem that leads to heart disease and stroke: a build-up of cholesterol and fat in the arteries. This condition is not only preventable through diet, it is even at least partially reversible. The primary cause of cardiovascular disease – clogged arteries in the heart and the brain – is too much saturated fat in the diet. Keep your intake of saturated fat low by cooking with small amounts of liquid oils, such as olive or canola oil. instead of margarine or butter and by minimizing your intake of fatty foods, such as full-fat mayonnaise, rich desserts and fatty meats.

Getting plenty of fruits and vegetables is also important. Fruits and vegetables are packed with antioxidants, compounds that block the effects of harmful oxygen molecules called free radicals. This is important because when free radicals damage the harmful low-density lipoprotein (LDL) cholesterol, it becomes stickier and more likely to stick to artery walls.

Studies have shown that antioxidants in fruits and vegetables can help prevent Alzheimer's disease. In 2002, researchers studied nearly 5,500 people and found that those who ate diets rich in antioxidants, vitamin C and E, lowered their risk of developing Alzheimer's disease Citrus fruits, kiwifruit, sprouts, broccoli, and cabbage are packed with vitamin C. While whole grains, nuts, milk and egg yolks contain vitamin E.

The combination of reducing fat in your diet and eating plenty of fruits and vegetables will help to keep your arteries clear, including those leading to your brain. In fact, it may even help restore blood flow through arteries that have already begun to close up.

Coffee can Improve Memory Function It's not without reason that millions of Americans jump start their day with steaming cups of coffee. The caffeine in coffee has been shown to improve mental functioning, including memory.

In one study, Dutch researchers used a chemical to block short-term memory in 16 healthy people. They found that giving these people 250 milligrams of caffeine – about the amount of 3 cups of coffee – quickly restored their powers of recall. However, too much coffee can be bad, if only the java buzz wears off within 6 to 8 hrs. For some people, at least, the after-coffee slump can result in mental fogginess.

Everyone has different reactions to caffeine. For people who rarely drink coffee, having a cup or two can definitely improve performance and memory. But if you drink coffee throughout the day, you quickly build up tolerance and you won't get the same benefits. In fact, too much caffeine can make you jittery and reduce your concentration.

Don't kill your brain cells "Killing brain cells is not the best way to get a high score in the memory department. Yet that's exactly what many of us do to our grey matter every day. Alcohol is drinking too much alcohol can cause a significant decrease in memory function." In fact, even small amounts of alcohol can damage cells in the brain responsible for memory.

Many doctors recommend abstaining from alcohol all together to keep your mind at its sharpest. At the very least, it's a good idea to limit yourself to one or two drinks – meaning 12 ounces of beer, 5 ounces of wine or 11/2 ounces of liquor – a day. When you do drink, choose red wine. It contains resveratrol, a compound that may keep your brain young.

Optimal Diet for your Brain You can't prevent Alzheimer's disease and dementia altogether, but you can keep them at bay longer with a heart-healthy diet that focuses on the nutrients that have been found to be critical for brain function and aging.

Aim for a body mass index of 23 to 25 Being overweight increases your risk for diabetes, metabolic syndrome, and hypertension, which leads to vascular disease and brain damage.

Choose Dairy Eat one serving of low-fat, low-sugar dairy once a day, such as milk, plain yogurt, cottage cheese or ricotta cheese. Epidemiologic studies show that people who drink milk are less likely to develop Alzheimer's disease.

Toast to a young brain Drink one glass of red wine or 4 ounces of purple grape juice or pomegranate juice a day. They contain resveratrol, a compound that doctors believe activates a gene that is associated with longevity.

Buy berries When you eat one cup of berries a day, it gives your brain resveratrol, and other flavonoids, that strengthens your resistance against the development of chronic diseases associated with aging.

Drink some juice Drink 8 ounces of fruit juice high in vitamin C daily. Three times a week, substitute a glass of vegetable juice that you buy or make on your own for the fruit juice. Antioxidants and other compounds in those juices help protect the brain from dementia.

Include fish oil in your diet. Omega-3 fatty acids are powerful agents for a healthy heart and arteries. When you eat oily cold-water fish such as sardines or mackerel you will ensure that you get enough omega-3. You can also substitute with 2,000 to 3,000 mg of fish oil or flaxseed oil per day. Walnuts are also rich in omega-3. Eating 8 to 10 walnuts per day or using walnut oil in your salads of dark green vegetables will help protect your brain.

Drink green tea every day. Green tea is rich in antioxidants and has proved to reduce the risk of dementia. Experts recommend drinking one to two cups a day.

Multivitamins To include those in your diet is particularly important for older, inactive adults whose calorie intake doesn't supply the micronutrients that they need. Choose a multivitamin without iron or reduced iron if you 're not anaemic or menstruating.

Consider supplementing with vitamin D Vitamin D is a new shining start in the role of brain development and function and many people are deficient without knowing it. We get about 95% of our vitamin D from sunlight, but young people who work long hours and elderly adults who are home bound often don't get enough sunlight to fill their vitamin D requirements.

Avoid omega-6 fats. Omega-6 fatty acids in corn- safflower- and sesame oils aren't as healthy as omega-3's found in olive and canola oil. So use those oils sparingly.

Nourish Your Brain An overall brain-healthy diet is low in refined carbohydrates, (Found in sugars, baked food, candy, and other sweets, for example), red meats and trans fats. It's high in fatty fish, poultry, soy protein, fruits, vegetables and legumes.

37. Sleepdisorders

There is nothing more beneficial than a good night sleep and there is a great physiological need for it if the individual likes to feel refreshed and alert during the following day. Sleep is also important for your memory and learning capacity and possibly for maintaining a good immune system. But there are still many unanswered questions regarding the function of sleep.

This is possibly best explained with the fact that people suffering from insomnia also suffer from reduced concentration, reduced memory and decreased ability to accomplish daily tasks. They are also at greater risk for work related accidents and road accidents, many sick days, increased use of healthcare services and a lower perceived quality of life.

Insomnia is usually perceived as related to not getting enough sleep, which means that the person either has trouble falling or staying asleep. However, poor quality of sleep, whereby the sufferer wakes up feeling unrefreshed, even after sufficient hours spent sleeping, is a common complaint, especially by elderly people.

Melatonin is a naturally occurring hormone in the brain, manufactured by the pineal gland and secreted at night. It is quickly degraded, but by being continuously secreted all through the night, it acts like a sleep regulator and 'signal of darkness' in humans. However, the natural production of melatonin tends to decrease with age. specially in elderly suffering from insomnia, the production of melatonin is decreased compared to elderly with no sleep problems.

Research has proven that melatonin, when taken in small doses of 0.1 milligram, can decrease the effects of jetlag, like sleeping difficulties and tiredness. The pill has to be taken just before bedtime on the place of destination and after arrival a few days, again just before going to bed.

Because melatonin is a natural product, it can be sold at the chemist in small concentrations of 0.1 milligram, wh20 has hardly any affect. You can't get addicted to melatonin and most people feel better during daytime.

Circadin, a sustained-release melatonin, is a new treatment paradigm in the management of primary insomnia in patients aged 55 years or over. A novel sleep drug, the first in a new class, Circadin provides natural sleep for patients with insomnia, offering an effective and save treatment for their sleep difficulties because it improves sleep quality, with a far superior safety and tolerability profile.

However, according to the authorities, circadin doesn't work equally effective for everybody,

Circadin contains 2 milligram of melatonin. Sleep occurs quicker with improved quality of life and better functionality during daytime.

References

CHAPTER 1

1. A Guide to Healthy Living
Dr Laz Bannock, PhD - Healthy Cells & Supplements
Dr Michael Colgan - Medicine for The Millennium - Acid-alkaline balance
Dr Ray D. Strand, M. D. - What Your Doctor doesn't know about nutritional may be killing you.

2. Nutrition: the key to Fitness and Well-being
Dr Myron Wentz - founder of USANA Health Sciences
Dr Laz Bannock, PhD - Healthy Cells & Supplements

3. Nutrition Facts
Dr Michael Colgan - Antioxidants against Disease
Dr Ray D. Strand, M.D. - Nutritional Medicine - Cellular nutrition
Dr Laz Bannock, PhD - Healthy Cells and Supplements

4. Good nutrition as part of a healthy lifestyle
Mike Geary - Fat Burning Kitchen

5. Preventive Medicine
Dr Ray D. Strand, M.D. - Preventive Medicine

6. Eat the right nutrients when aging
The Doctors Book of Food Remedies by Selene Yeager
and the Editors of Prevention - Aging

CHAPTER #2

7. Healthy for Life with Natural Digestive Enzymes
The Doctors Book of Food Remedies by Selene Yeager
and the Editors of Prevention - Phytonutrients

8. Eating Healthy - the GI Way
USANA.com
thefactsaboutfitness.com/articles/glycemic index
The Glycemic Index & Glycemic Load - mendosa.com

9. Vitamin D deficiency
USANA Health Sciences

10. Synergy in vitamin & mineral supplementation
Dr Michael Colgan - The New Nutrition
Osteoporosis is epidemic
USANA Health Sciences

11. A healthy brain diet prevent stroke
Dr Michael Colgan - The New Nutrition
Save Your Brain
The Doctors Book of Food Remedies by Selene Yeager
Memory Problems

12. How food effects our mood
The Doctors Book of Food Remedies by Selene Yeager
Memory problems

13. Benefits of a ketogenic diet
www.nutrobalance2.net

14. The Benefits of raw food
Dr Edward Howell - Food Enzymes for Health & Longevity

32. How to avoid chemicals at home
USANA Health Sciences

33. Problems concerning the heart
Dr Ray D. Strand, M.D - What Your Doctor doesn't know
about Nutritional Medicine MAY BE KILLING YOU
Chapter 7 Cardiomyopathy: New Hope for a Cure

34. How to overcome menopausal problems
Dr Mirkin.com
Dr Gabe Mirkin on exercise, health & nutrition

35. Prevention of memory problems
The Doctors Book of Food Remedies by Selene Yeager

36. Sleep disorders
http://www.lundbeck.com/products/our_products/circadin

About the Author

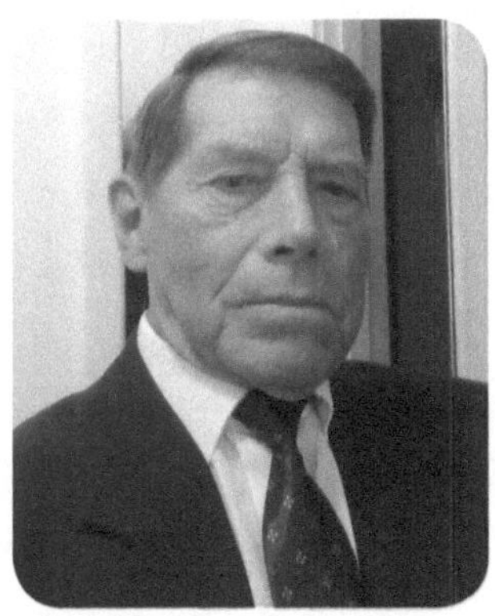

In 2008, I became an associate with a nutritional supplement manufacturer.

From that time on, I became more aware of the advantages of healthy living and a healthy lifestyle.

I heard about the bad eating habits of many Americans, which causes obesity, overweight, and degenerative diseases.

Since 2008, I wrote several articles about nutrition and weight loss and achieved expert status with EzineArticles.com. I have been involved in nutrition and weight management for more than twelve years.

In 2009, I created my own website and blog and called it Nutrobalance, which means balanced nutrition. Also, when I worked for this nutritional supplement company, I became aware of the importance of good nutrition.

I learned that it is true when they say, 'You are what you eat.' And you can add at least ten more years to your life by eating the right way and taking regular exercise.

When I moved to Australia in 1971, I gave up smoking and started swimming in the ocean every morning and played tennis quite regularly. In my later years, I practiced yoga, and also, since 2014, I started weightlifting, which is good for the bone structure. I really feel at least ten years younger.

I like to help people with weight management to improve their health and to create more awareness of the importance of a healthy lifestyle.

The reason I wrote this book is to provide the tools and the knowledge to maintain a healthy body by supplying the right exercises for aerobics and weight-bearing exercises, which are both important to maintain a healthy weight.

It is the author's desire that many people, young and old, will benefit from the content of this book.

Adrian Joele